THE RESILIENT
WRITERWHEELS

THE RESILIENT WRITERWHEELS
Can't is a bad word

ERIN M. KELLY

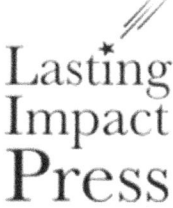
Lasting Impact Press

Pontiac, Illinois

Copyright Erin M. Kelly, 2020

All rights reserved. No portion nor the whole of this book may be reproduced or used whatsoever without written permission from the publisher except in the case of a brief quote included in reviews or critical articles. For information regarding licensing this content, or to order in bulk, write to Connection Victory Publishing Company P.O. Box 563, Pontiac, Illinois 61764-0563 or <info@connectionvictory.com> or use the contact form on our website: www.ConnectionVictory.com

Author: Erin M. Kelly

Editor: Wilhelm Cortez

Photos: Christie Clancy of Clancy214 Photography

***

Publisher's Cataloging-in-Publication Data provided by
Five Rainbows Cataloging Services

Names: Kelly, Erin M., author.

Title: The resilient writerwheels : can't is a bad word / Erin M. Kelly.

Description: Pontiac, IL : Lasting Impact Press, 2020.

Identifiers: ISBN 978-1-64381-026-3 (paperback) | ISBN 978-1-64381-027-0 (Kindle ebook)

Subjects: LCSH: Cerebral palsy--Biography. | People with disabilities--Biography. | Perseverance (Ethics) | Women authors--Biography. | Autonomy (Psychology) | BISAC: BIOGRAPHY & AUTOBIOGRAPHY / People with Disabilities. | SELF-HELP / Personal Growth / Success. | BIOGRAPHY & AUTOBIOGRAPHY / Personal Memoirs. | BIOGRAPHY & AUTOBIOGRAPHY / Women.

Classification: LCC RC388 .K45 2020 (print) | LCC RC388 (ebook) | DDC 616.8/360092--dc23.

Praise for *The Resilient WriterWheels*

Erin Kelly's *The Resilient WriterWheels* is a journey. Her life is in itself a journey through the intricate and often very difficult world of the life we are given, and how we allow our world around us to be shaped by our faith through that journey. She is a writer who has seen far more difficulties than many, but unlike many, has used those limitations in her life to make our world and hers better. To see that life on the pages of a book is an honor. Her book brings us into her world where she moves through the challenges of her young life, and in bringing us along, she both inspires and empowers us to glean from her, and to love her, and to find ourselves in her words.

This is a beautiful book about overcoming, about learning to own the world we are given, and turning that world into something far better than we had imagined. Every painful word, every painful memory of her life recorded in this book gives the reader the power to live our journey, no matter how hard or how easy it is for us. Erin Kelly is the embodiment of her story, the embodiment of her strength, and it is the subtlety of the strength and inspiration she brings us into as we journey with her in this book that make us gain her strength. I am honored to know her, to follow her journey, and to walk along as I read each word and connect her words to the writer that she is. The story teaches us that it is not how long or how difficult or how rough the journey is, but in how that journey shapes what we finally become. This is a powerful story from a powerful and necessary voice.

— ***Patricia Jabbeh Wesley***, *Author of* Praise Song for My Children: New and Selected Poems; *Professor of English, Creative Writing and African Lit, Penn State Altoona*

A Note From the Publisher

We're breaking convention to reduce blank pages.

In the book publishing industry, including among organizations such as the Independent Book Publishers Association, of which Connection Victory Publishing Company is a member, there is a convention that dictates a new chapter should be on the *recto* or right page of a print book. When following this standard, if the previous chapter ends on a recto, then the following *verso* or left page remains blank. In a book with many chapters, following this convention creates many blank pages, which is neither cost-effective nor environmentally sound.

For that reason, I have chosen to format this book such that Chapters 2 through 51 begin on the next full page, whether verso or recto. In the frontmatter, I have made only minimal adjustments to conserve pages.

While I understand that many book lovers prefer the conventional format, the result of my decision has eliminated 20 blank pages of paper from this print edition. As a reminder, paper comes from trees, and deforestation for the paper industry has contributed to our climate crisis.

Those of us who love our libraries of print books have to do what we can to reduce waste where we can. Thank you for allowing me to break from convention in this manner.

Lisa M. Blacker
President & Publisher
Connection Victory Publishing Company

THE RESILIENT
WRITERWHEELS

Erin M. Kelly
Writing Career Highlights

2009--Hired at The Altoona Mirror for a monthly column "The View From Here"

2010--Began editing the memoir *To Cope and To Prevail* by Dr. Ilse Rose Warg

2010--My poem "A Long Way from Hello" was published in Oberon Poetry Magazine

2012--Hired by Cameron Conaway as a Social Justice writer/contributor for The Good Men Project

2012--Completed editing process for *To Cope and To Prevail*, with my name listed in the book as Editor

2014--Hired as a writer at The Huffington Post

2014--My work was published by Wordgathering: A Journal of Disability Poetry and Literature for the first time

2014--Had numerous articles published by The Mighty

2014--Accepted a position as Social Justice Editor at The Good Men Project

2015--Wrote a blurb/review of John C. Mannone's book of poetry entitled *Disabled Monsters;* it was published on the back cover of his book.

2016--Hired as a contributor for Upworthy

2016--My work was published by XoJane

2016--Recognized as Top 20 Under 40/Altoona Mirror

2017--Work published by Breath and Shadow Journal

2018--My first book (poetry), *How To Wait*, was published by Finishing Line Press

2018--Wrote a review/blurb for Cameron Conaway's *Man Box: Poems* published by Lasting Impact Press, an imprint of Connection Victory Publishing Company

2018--Received WISE Women of Blair County Award in Arts and Letters

2019--My essay "Reluctant Reliance" was published in the anthology *Bodies of Truth: Personal Narratives on Illness, Disability, and Medicine*

2020--Acknowledged in Patricia Jabbeh Wesley's *Praise Song For My Children: New and Selected Poems*

2020—*The Resilient WriterWheels*: Can't Is a Bad Word, my autobiography is published by Lasting Impact Press, an imprint of Connection Victory Publishing Company

Follow Erin M. Kelly

Subscribe to learn more about Erin M. Kelly and her writing projects, use the QR code below or use this link:

http://bit.ly/ResilientWriterWheels

Social Media:

Facebook: https://www.facebook.com/WriterWheels/

Twitter: https://twitter.com/WriterWheels

About the Author

Erin M. Kelly was born with cerebral palsy and wants to be recognized for her work rather than her disability. She enjoys writing in all genres and has been published by The Huffington Post, Upworthy, The Mighty, The Good Men Project, and others. Her essay, "Reluctant Reliance" is featured in the anthology, *Bodies of Truth: Personal Essays on Illness, Disability, and Medicine*. Erin served as Editor for the memoir, *To Cope and To Prevail*, by Dr. Ilse-Rose Warg. She also writes a monthly column entitled, "The View From Here," for the local newspaper in Altoona, Pennsylvania, addressing the challenges she faces daily. Erin is the author of *How To Wait*, her debut collection of poetry. *The Resilient WriterWheels: Can't Is a Bad Word* is her autobiography.

Dedication

I dedicate this book to every person who has ever read anything I've written at any point in my career, and to those who support my journey by continuing to read my work. You are the reason why I'm still on this path.

Acknowledgments

I would like to express my constant, deeply heartfelt gratitude to the countless professionals in the writing and publishing industry, from editors to my personal mentors, who have helped guide me through my career and navigate the tough, relentless routine that comes with being a writer. Without you, my dream to do this for a living would have remained just that -- a dream.

A special acknowledgment goes out to Wilhelm Cortez, my Editor at The Good Men Project and the guiding hand behind this autobiography. I've always wanted see how far I could go as a writer, and you've given me to encouragement and freedom to truly spread my wings. Thank you for believing in me and my ambitious imagination!

Introduction

Writing To Feel Free and Understood

Honesty is the gift writing allows me to share.

The expression "Walk a mile in someone else's shoes" has always meant a lot to me. It speaks directly to my soul, not because I'm physically unable to walk, but instead because I take it to heart. As a kid, I became angry when I heard those words. I felt as if no one truly knew what it's like to have cerebral palsy, no matter how hard they tried to understand the disability itself. More importantly, they didn't understand me.

Now, as an adult, I would be a fool to convince myself that I don't still feel that way. What's worse, however, is the gut feeling that some people are not fully willing to think or comprehend things in a different way, unless they absolutely have to. My saving grace has been writing. I've been writing for as long as I can remember. It didn't matter whether I was scribbling with a crayon or trying to deal with my cerebral palsy in my own way. When I wrote, I felt free and understood.

That feeling never left or grew old. In fact, it has laid the foundation for my career as a columnist, journalist, and poet. Most importantly, my personal need to be understood has allowed me to be honest with myself and anyone who reads my work. That's one of the things that my many years of writing has given me. If writing does nothing else for me, I'll be forever grateful for the gift of honesty it continually allows me to share. As time passes and my career grows, I realize there's no shame in putting that on display.

I'm equally grateful that my writing has allowed other people to be honest with me, whether about my disability or how my work inspires them. I never know how anything I write will be received by those who read it, but I have to take risks and always hope for the best. With that being said, the story you're about to read is authentically mine. My words. My thoughts.

Some parts of this book are written out of my unwavering willingness to be brutally honest. Some of it comes from very dark corners in my mind, and there are others that I'm admittedly not proud of. This is the first time I've written my story in its entirety. It's also a reflection of the incredible opportunity I've had to motivate or inspire others in some small way over the years.

At first, growing up in the small town of Altoona, Pennsylvania, I didn't see much opportunity to thrive as a writer with cerebral palsy. I always thought that people went to work---regardless of whether or not they enjoyed what they were doing---to make ends meet. I didn't realize I could do something I love and still make a positive impact, until things slowly began happening for me on a professional level.

To everyone reading this book: I hope it leaves you with something worthwhile. I hope it gives you a reason to be open to thinking differently. I hope it inspires you in some way.

Table of Contents

Praise for The Resilient WriterWheels..v

A Note From the Publisher..vi

Erin M. Kelly Writing Career Highlights...viii

Follow Erin M. Kelly..x

About the Author..xi

Dedication..xii

Acknowledgments..xiii

Introduction: Writing To Feel Free and Understood...................xiv

Table of Contents..xvi

Chapter 1: Warning: A Storm Is Coming......................................1

Chapter 2: Abilities Outshine Disability..5

Chapter 3: Acceptance Is a Delicate Thread of Humanity.........8

Chapter 4: Some Barriers Don't Block Friends..........................11

Chapter 5: The Never-Ending Maze of Life 14

Chapter 6: Perception, Adoption, and Identity 18

Chapter 7: Growing Up Around Men 22

Chapter 8: When Time Reveals the Ugly Truth 26

Chapter 9: Laugh Off the Wall 29

Chapter 10:
> How To Get the Goal When You Have To Go Back..........32

Chapter 11: When Frustration Occurs Again and Again 36

Chapter 12: How To Use What You Have.................39

Chapter 13: The Measure of Maturity....................42

Chapter 14: Age Has a Funny Way of Changing Your Life 45

Chapter 15: Dangerous, Delicate Power..................49

Chapter 16: How To Develop a Quiet Respect.............53

Chapter 17: Mutual Respect Showdown..................56

Chapter 18: Trust Your Gut............................60

Chapter 19: Mindsets Change To Rise Above the Negative ...64

Chapter 20:
> Life Throws Curveballs When We Least Expect It 68

Chapter 21: There Are Days When Time Stands Still............72

Chapter 22: Where Are the Loyal?......................76

Chapter 23: What Is a Worthwhile Moment?.............80

Chapter 24: Realize the Potential......................84

Chapter 25: Take a Chance on Yourself.................88

Chapter 26: There's a Time and a Place for Everything..........91

Chapter 27: Center the Inner Force 95

Chapter 28: Lift Another and Elevate Yourself...............98

Chapter 29: Burdens To Bear 101

Chapter 30: Momentum Motivates 104

Chapter 31:
  Dig Deep and Drown the Noise the World Makes 107

Chapter 32: Don't Let Them Tear You Down 111

Chapter 33: Finding the Strength To Let Go 115

Chapter 34: Bounce Back 119

Chapter 35: The Clock Doesn't Stop 123

Chapter 36: Represent Yourself and Let It Out 127

Chapter 37: Accomplishment on Your Own Terms 130

Chapter 38: What Paths Life Takes 133

Chapter 39: The Lies in Our Goodbyes 137

Chapter 40: Vulnerability Is a Scary Kind of Magic 141

Chapter 41: When the Stars Align, or Don't 146

Chapter 42: What's Worthwhile to You? 149

Chapter 43: Respect Rolls the Dice 153

Chapter 44: Be the Moment 156

Chapter 45:
  The Fine Line Between Integrity and Self-Care 160

Chapter 46: Appreciate the Process 164

Chapter 47: Create the Inclusive for Yourself 168

Chapter 48: Up and Down the Peaks in the Valley 172

Chapter 49: Crawl Out of Your Hole 177

Chapter 50: Dreams and Truth 182

Chapter 51: There Are Mountains To Move 187

Forthcoming by Erin M. Kelly... 192

Previously Published Components... 193

Index... 198

Also Published by Lasting Impact Press, An Imprint of
  Connection Victory Publishing Company........................ 201

Chapter 1

Warning: A Storm Is Coming

When patience is not an option.

There's a storm coming. I can feel it deep in my bones. This storm—my storm—comes like a thief who tries in the night to steal the crown jewel of my soul: my inner peace. The sun isn't shining through my window blinds yet, so I roll over in my bed and wipe the sleep from my eyes. To my left, I see the most enduring figure in my life, my wheelchair, parked a few feet from my bed. It's a constant, sharp reminder of my cerebral palsy—one of the most common disabilities known to man that can affect everything from brain function to fine motor skills needed for tying a pair of shoelaces or brushing one's teeth.

I pull my bed-sheet up far enough to cover my legs, while grudgingly asking myself why I'm so patient and why it's such a virtue before switching my gaze over to my right. My shrine to one of my biggest heroes, Dwayne 'The Rock' Johnson, brings an automatic smile to my face because it's a measure of happiness and, in some ways, redemption for the many times I've fought a quiet war against myself and won.

I wait for a parade of early morning footsteps to pass over the threshold of the wheelchair-accessible entrance of my room before I enter my always busy household. One long, slow breath while I remind myself that nothing is a simple case of mind over matter when it comes to doing basic, everyday things.

I look around at my cotton candy pink walls and laugh out loud because I don't like to allow myself to become consumed by my circumstances or the situations they put me in—situations where I have to wait even more than I already do. Outside my door, I hear my family rattle off their itinerary for the day:

"I have to go to the store."

"I have to stop at the bank after work."

Then the storm hits.

That's the moment when the ever-present storm inside me begins to rage, and I'm forced to put the very attribute I wish I didn't have into use. It takes all I have to lay there and listen when all I want to do is get up and move with the same flow as the rest of my family.

But. I. Can't.

The flow and coordination aren't there—because it isn't mine, and I don't pretend it is mine.

There's a certain degree of inner peace in knowing I have my own flow as a habitual thinker and, most importantly, as a writer—the same way a painter or a sculptor has theirs. It doesn't change the fact that I'm disabled, or the amount of patience required for me to live my life the way I want to live it. I think I embrace my flow to its fullest because I had to search long and hard to find it. It wasn't given to me in a neatly wrapped package, but now that I've found it, I've made a promise to myself to always protect it.

For me, having patience isn't a choice, nor is it something I've particularly wanted to master.

In truth, having patience is a lesson I would much rather have learned in my own time or by my own hand, but the cards weren't dealt to me in that manner.

I find myself waiting for everything from getting dressed to getting into a car. Getting into a car means surrendering to someone else whatever freedom I have and giving in to doing things their way, on their time. I can't even begin to describe how much my patience has been tested in that regard, so I won't try to make up some riveting story about it.

How ironic that my cerebral palsy strangely encompasses the vastness of Webster's Dictionary, which defines patience as "the capacity, habit or fact of being patient." To simply take that at face value would be the easy thing to do—as well as the expected thing to do because we all have to wait for something at some point in our lives. Some might argue that you only need to have patience in certain situations in life, while others can be somewhat rushed.

In fact, "the capacity, habit or fact of being patient" seems like a very broad definition for a word that can carry so much weight and emotion. Yet patience itself is so much more than just a word, particularly in today's world. Patience is a practice some can get good at or even master. If patience is defined by such simple principles, I think it's only fair that every human being has the right to apply them to their lives however they see fit—or at least try to.

It doesn't mean it's right or wrong.

It's about finding ways to live on one's own terms, regardless of how difficult the journey may be.

I find living with cerebral palsy—while also having an abundance of forced patience—is a habit as well as a cold, hard fact, just like Webster's Dictionary says. I struggle to find the capacity to grasp this notion: I can't get myself out of bed in the morning, but I can write a 1600-word story or article without thinking twice. That's just a small piece of the puzzle when I stop and think about all the things I have to wait for on a daily basis. Somehow, it still only scratches the surface.

All I know is there's a very delicate balance to all of this—a balance I'm immensely grateful to have found for the sake of my sanity. It's something I had to find on my own, or I never would have known what it truly means to always be honest with myself about needing help… and having to wait to get it. I've learned to accept the fact that while I may not like having patience, my disability demands it.

There are no two ways about it. It's not the way I choose to be. It's the way I have to be.

At the end of the day, I have to remind myself that I didn't ask for any of this. I didn't cause this storm. I just happen to be in the middle of it every day. This is my life, and I still wake up and face the day with fire in my heart and a smile on my face!

Chapter 2

Abilities Outshine Disability

Yet, I will always have something to prove.

We all come to a crossroad at some point. We're caught between drifting away from who we are and being pulled back in. When we weigh the pros and cons, choosing both may be good for us.

I came to my crossroad when I was ten or eleven years old. Writing was the essential piece of my life that had been missing for what seemed like forever. It allowed me to express myself in ways my disability didn't. Writing made me happy, but I still had so much to prove.

Moving forward with life required that I show the world I wasn't emotionally attached to my disabled label. The trick was finding an effective way to put myself out there. I had a strong feeling writing was eventually going to do that. However, I hated the fact I had to prove myself just because people looked at me a certain way.

I didn't have a clue where to begin to polish the words I wrote. Nor did I know any writers at the time. All I had was a burning desire to be understood—and a dream to one day become the writer I always told my parents I wanted to be. There were days when I wanted to crawl into a corner and wait to deal with all of this until I was ready. I knew the need to prove myself was never going away. Part of me thought life would get a little easier after I did.

A tiny voice in my head tried to convince me that every person I'd ever cross paths with wouldn't see my wheelchair before they saw *me*. It wasn't long before I realized how naive I was to think this, even as nice and calming as it may have been. People were still questioning my abilities into my early teen years. I still did my best to use their doubts as motivation. I heard them begin to whisper, or talk under their breath because they thought I wasn't listening. Even more degrading, people got in my face and started talking loudly—like I couldn't hear or didn't understand what they were saying.

That made me go out of my way to show everyone the pictures I drew, the mess I'd made while playing with silly putty or whatever creation I could put my stamp on. I showed them off because they were mine, and I wanted others to see that my abilities outshone my disability.

Sometimes, I would get a faint smile of approval from strangers before they walked away. There wasn't much beyond that. I started to wonder why I was expected to give so much of myself when some people didn't even notice.

So, I did what any kid would do. I turned to my mom and asked her, "Why do I always have to prove myself?"

She looked at me with quiet confidence and said, "You're going to have to prove yourself for the rest of your life, Erin. This is the way it has to be."

That was the end of the conversation. My mom's voice was soft but stern at that moment. I never asked the question again, because I didn't need to. I knew this was the beginning of the rest of my days—as a human being, writer and everything else I hoped to be. This conversation wasn't the only one I'd have about my disability. It was, however, the first one that stuck with me.

As an adult, I realize I don't have everything figured out. Nor have I felt everything there is to feel. As more emotions slowly become tangled with my circumstances, there will be more conversations. More emotions to wrestle with. I might be able to keep them at bay for a while, but they'll always be there just below the surface.

I know I will always have something to prove. There will always be someone who will see my shadow first.

Chapter 3

Acceptance Is a Delicate Thread of Humanity

Self acceptance is a path to the acceptance of others as they are.

I thought I'd cause a rip or tear if I contributed to the fabric of society. I had come to a comfortable place of acceptance where doing everyday things proved to be a major feat. Then, I was suddenly blinded by the uncomfortable glow of uncertainty.

My entire life, I've been put underneath a microscope but have never needed to ask why. I watch as people walk by while their eyes ask the questions their lips don't dare. A familiar chill runs down my spine because I know most don't see me first. They see my wheelchair and the label that comes with it.

Part of me doesn't blame those who silently interrogate me. Another part of me secretly despises the automatic connection made between my disability and how it simultaneously gives others a scale to gauge my abilities.

That connection is usually based on the fact that I look meek, mild, and almost feeble on the surface. I wish it wasn't that way, but I'm well aware of the label placed on me. It's my personal responsibility to decide how I wear that label because it, in turn, determines how I'm treated.

That's the primary reason why I will put my heart and soul into everything I will ever do. It's not because I strive to be liked or even admired, nor because I was raised to always find a way to make things work. It's because I want to eventually be accepted and to do everything I can to carve out a place in society for myself.

In the eyes of those who simply write me off, I might not look like I know exactly what's going on around me. They're likely not going to see that I'm very observant and probably know too much for my own good. They're not going to take note of the fact I'm adopted from Korea, either. It has admittedly taken me many years to be OK with all of this, which has helped me become more accepting of people who don't share my beliefs and viewpoints.

I've found the people who are willing to ask me questions are the same ones who are willing to accept me for who I am. They acknowledge the label I wear as a badge of honor without calling obvious attention to it. There's no better feeling in the world than that!

My shadow is much bigger than my body. It's difficult for some people to see anything else. It's hard for me to wrap my head around that because I've always tried not to limit my view of the world. I may not be able to leave my shadow behind, but I try my best to quietly shed the weight it puts on my shoulders.

That is what makes me different. When I came to understand the ways of my own world, I knew I had my personal mission. I never want to give anyone a reason to believe I'm "the girl in a wheelchair." If anything, I hope to change some minds. I know how I want to be seen.

I find my place in society by learning to adapt to my circumstances and writing about my experiences. This is something worthwhile. It gives people a reason to pause—and perhaps think, 'Hey, this woman knows what she's doing. Maybe we were wrong.'

When my world gets heavy, the power of writing and living my truth always brings me to a better place. It has become my gateway to true and full acceptance and opened the door for those who may be standing outside waiting for the right time to knock. So, will you come in?

Chapter 4

Some Barriers Don't Block Friends

Meaningful friendships are worth waiting for amid all the distractions.

What a strange feeling it is to be young and not know which way is the right way. On top of all that, add having a disability, which brings necessity into focus in the blink of an eye.

I shifted my attention to things other than my cerebral palsy. This was one big step out of my comfort zone during my adolescence and early teenage years because I was still wrestling with floods of emotion while trying to figure out who I truly was.

Was this the sum of my existence? I was getting older and wanted to see what else the world had to offer---a huge transition out of my comfort zone. I'd been going to school for half-days in a special inclusion class with other kids who had disabilities. It was the first time I can remember being around people who truly didn't understand me.

I didn't know them and they didn't know me. Everyone feels awkward when they're around someone they don't know.

However, it was much deeper than the feeling of simply being in the company of complete strangers.

Their stares penetrated my bones. I knew they were looking at the obvious: my wheelchair, my body. It was nothing new, but I still wanted to make the most of this new adventure. I would show off the smile I had learned to flash whenever I would met new people. If anything, I wanted to try to make some friends. I just hoped my classmates wouldn't single me out. If I didn't end up making any friends here, maybe I could meet new ones somewhere else.

Making friends proved to be less painful and embarrassing than I thought it would be. No one called me out or made fun of me. Everyone was more interested in the communication board I'd gotten to help me "speak" better as I got older. The other kids gathered around my wheelchair and tried their best to restrain from pressing all the buttons on the board. It lit up every time I pressed one of the 140 keys. They understood, for the most part, that I had the board because it helped me. They knew it was a part of who I was, even though I was apprehensive about having another thing to distract people from looking at me.

The communication board provided the ultimate freedom the first time I used it. Every thought and feeling I had locked up inside me finally had a way out. The one thing my classmates didn't realize was that each key stood for three or four different words and phrases. One wrong hit could've wiped out the entire system that had been specifically programmed for me.

It felt good knowing other people were starting to understand why I needed that board, and why it wasn't a "toy".

I'd gotten good at using it, even learned to type with a little speed. However, it wasn't helping me make any real friends.

I understood curiosity comes with my territory, so I didn't mind all of the excitement that came with my communication board. I did, however, mind the automated male RoboCop voice it was programmed with. I already felt strange about the fact it would likely draw more attention to my disability. Now, I had to somehow hide my embarrassment every time I "spoke".

Most people didn't care, but I did. I eventually asked for my "voice" to be changed to a female one. It was more about trying to show other kids that it was OK to be friends with me than anything else. I never wanted to allow my needs as a disabled person to get in the way of any potential friendships—and having a male voice didn't seem like a good way to introduce myself to people.

Making that small change opened the door for many more. It gave me a sense of normalcy in many ways. It made me realize I was a kid who had to grow up. Maybe not in the conventional way most kids do but I had to do it, eventually. This particular moment was a pretty good start.

I've since "graduated" from using my communication board and now have true, meaningful friendships with people from all walks of life. It has taken a very long me to grow and learn from this. The most important lesson it has taught me is: Though it may take a while, the best things in life are truly worth the wait!

Chapter 5

The Never-Ending Maze of Life

Are you willing to adapt and level the playing field?

The world is an intricate, never-ending maze. Every twist and turn is a reason to question one's own sanity while trying to find ways to adapt, and, sometimes, conquer. There may be a way out but it doesn't look like a way out at first. Getting lost isn't real until all apparent paths have been rendered useless.

From a very early age, I've found myself in the middle of this maze of effectively living the life I've been given. That has meant learning how to strategically place a fork and spoon in between my fingers to feed myself, figuring out how to turn on a light switch, and navigating my wheelchair through a narrow doorway without ripping the frame off. All of these everyday things, among others, proved to be monumental tasks at one point or another in my life due to cerebral palsy.

When I did these small tasks, no matter how long it took or how awkward I looked, I was fulfilled in a very personal sense. I was simultaneously learning to play an instrument and perfecting a dance routine every time I figured out an effective way of doing something. That is the hard truth of living with a disability. I'd be wrong if I didn't try to do what I need to do to be comfortable in my own skin while being fully aware that able-bodied individuals do many of the same things I do every day—just at a more fluent, quicker pace.

However, that doesn't stop me from trying to figure things out for myself.

I do simple, everyday tasks a hundred times over—not because I like doing them, but because I usually have difficulty due to my lack of speed or physical limitations. I always try to discover a trick to be able to do something on my own, or with little assistance.

By the same token, I also try to keep in mind that most people don't have my set of circumstances. They might not have to think about the width of a doorway, the height of a curb or if they can reach their bed sheets to pull up on a cold night. I respect the fact these thoughts likely never cross people's minds. At the same time, however, I hope others respect that I do think about little things like these because they help me determine how I live my life.

There's something incredibly invigorating about using my own brain and two hands to accomplish something. I can guarantee it won't be perfect or flowing in a steady rhythm like the way I envision it in my mind's eye, but it will be done. I'm constantly chasing the feeling of personal accomplishment—and admittedly, I love when it rushes through my body to my fingertips.

The process isn't always pretty or smooth.

There's a lot of trial and error involved. It could be as simple as brushing my teeth one day. The next day, however, it might be something more complicated—like plugging my phone into my computer so it can charge. Both tasks require both of my hands, so my mind goes to a place where all I'm focused on is that toothbrush or that cord. Ten, twenty minutes later, the mission is accomplished—but not without acknowledging exactly what it took.

I adapt to whatever situation I'm in because I genuinely don't know any other way to function. I've accepted that I'm often not able to do things the way other people do them—the way they're supposed to be done. The feeling radiates all the way down to my toes, and I don't expect anyone reading this to understand how powerless and draining it truly is.

Most of the things I do on a daily basis take a lot of my time and energy, which is probably why I'm so patient. I know for some people, that might not seem noteworthy because everything takes time—no matter who you are or what your situation is. I also know, however, that if I don't adapt to my disability, it will take over and run my life.

As I get older, I realize I'm more honed in on adapting my perspectives about my disability from the sheer fact that it affects every single aspect of my existence. From the way I eat to the way I scout out handicapped parking spaces while a designated driver is at the wheel. That's an incredibly bitter pill to swallow, but it's small compared to the view I've grown accustomed to while sitting in my chair.

I imagine others might have to adjust their view when they step into my world. Instead of looking down, they'd have to be willing to look up because everything is bigger and taller when sitting down. They'd also have to be willing to adapt and level the playing field—not just for themselves, but for everyone.

I really want people to feel like they could jump into my world and feel what it's like to have society pass you by, to think they don't have a voice or a place in my universe. In truth, they definitely do have a place here. In my world, no possibility is deemed "useless" because I wouldn't have the life and career I have if every path were a straight line leading to comfort, success, and most importantly, peace of mind.

Life doesn't come with a blueprint. It doesn't come with a way to escape the maze. Life gave me a reason to find my own way—and I'm so grateful it did!

Chapter 6

Perception, Adoption, and Identity

What are you going to do with the words I can't?

Perception is a beautifully powerful tool if it's not misused. Everything looks clear if it's not cracked or shattered from the moment opinions are formed and views begin to change.

This is the best time to truly evaluate oneself and try to make things as perfect as they can be. Very few aspects of my life have been flawless, and they likely never will be. Everyone has things in their lives they can't take back or change. You get to a point where you can accept your personal truth. However, there are always other things about life that demand the same kind of attention.

It had become pretty clear that my perception and views were nothing like those of the people around me. It was a burning feeling in my gut and something I couldn't hide. I couldn't cover up the fact that I'm adopted from Seoul, Korea. That would've meant hiding my face, my body and perhaps most importantly, the other half of my identity as seen by the rest of the world.

Korean was my identity as an abandoned 10-month old coming to the U.S.—and it always will be. I didn't want that to be "swept under the rug". It was, and still is, just as important to my story as my disability is.

I was adopted into a devoted and hard-working family in the small railroad town of Altoona, Pennsylvania after my dad stumbled upon my picture in a pamphlet about adoption. He noticed part of the caption said, "...has cerebral palsy" and anxiously called my mom, who worked in a special needs program at the time, to ask what it was.

With a son already adopted from Korea, my parents were determined to do everything they could to adopt me. It took many sleepless nights and disconnected flights to JFK Airport in New York City to do so, but they were headstrong enough to see it through. It's difficult for me to articulate how grateful I am they didn't give up, because they easily could have. I wouldn't have the life I have if they hadn't persisted. Nor would I be able to write about this if it weren't for the selflessness of my birth mother—whom I've never met.

My parents haven't looked back since adopting me, and neither have I. I stopped questioning a lot of things when I was old enough to understand this part of my life. I didn't have anything solid to fall back on, so my adoption was all I knew. In my mind, it was always where my story started. There was no lucrative trail of information leading up to my birth. The only tangible detail I remember my parents telling me is that I was left in a police station in Korea with a note that read, "Please adopt her to a family that can raise her."

As young as I was, I didn't want to forget that—ever. I also didn't want the fact I am adopted to scare people away, especially anyone who potentially wanted to be my friend.

Yes, everyone could see I already had a very large, overwhelming shadow. Everyone questioned it, but no one seemed to stare at my jet-black hair, oriental eyes, and lightly-tanned skin the way they stared at my wheelchair as I got older.

It seemed no one was as willing to ask questions about my adoption when I was a kid—unless my parents initiated the conversation. People thought there was a big, mysterious correlation between my adoption and diagnosis of cerebral palsy. So, when they did ask questions, they would say things like, "Did you have to pay for her because she has a disability?" All the while, there I was—sitting in a stroller beside my older brother.

My parents always smiled and politely replied, "No, we worked very hard to get our children. We love them, and we treat our daughter like any other child."

My parents initially decided not to tell many family members about my diagnosis. They hoped the rest of the family would accept my disability for what it was—and not look at me with pity. Little did they know, they would get their wish in a beautiful, unexpected way.

During an adoption seminar, our local newscaster decided to do the news with me on her lap. My mom frantically called my grandparents to tell them about my cerebral palsy so they didn't find out on the newscast. My grandfather's voice was filled with joy as he said, "I knew she was special!"

I was raised to always try and go beyond what's expected. I couldn't have been brought up any other way with parents who worked night shifts in restaurants and offices and grandparents who were dirt poor. The ramifications of my diagnosis were that I was "supposed" to only go so far in life before I'd reach a certain capacity. In fact, I wasn't allowed to say, "I can't", but rather, "I'll try."

I wasn't supposed to have this life, but I'm here. And thriving. I'm showing everyone what I've done with the words, I can't. The question is, *What will* you *do with them?*

Chapter 7

Growing Up Around Men

Sometimes, you need to put your head down, get your hands dirty, and get things done.

We become attached to certain people or things. The reasons can be emotional, physical, or intellectual. Whatever they may be, we have to own them. They help shape who we are.

I wasn't attached to material things as a baby. I didn't need a teddy bear or a blanket before I went to sleep. The usual pre-planned car rides did the trick, as I'd bawl my eyes out for hours on end. It was nothing for me to continue crying for 12 hours straight. My cerebral palsy didn't calm me down at all; it only intensified my outbursts of tears. The longer I cried, the more my diagnosis came into effect.

I was more attached to the men in my family than anything or anyone else. My bond with them was immediate and genuine. I don't know where it came from, but my mom has always attributed it to the fact that I had two male escorts when I came to the U.S. from Korea. My attraction to men was so strong and evident that I'd burst in tears when the female flight attendant on the plane held me or came near me.

It proved to be a very strong, dominant trait I had that made for many, many long, loud sleepless nights (and days) for my mom. She often needed a break from my "episodes" as she desperately tried everything she could think of to get me to sleep or, even better, to stop crying. She'd even sit in a chair and rock back and forth with me in her arms until her body went limp.

Nothing she did soothed me, so she would call my dad or grandfather in hopes of getting a few minutes of peace and quiet. It worked. There was dead silence the second I heard one of their voices on the other end of the phone. They'd talk to me for five or ten minutes and I was fine.

It was as if someone had flipped a switch. It provided a much-needed distraction for my mom, who was beyond exhausted. This also gave me few moments of comfort. As soon as she hung up that phone, however, the cycle started all over again.

When my grandfather came over to our house, as he'd often do, he held and cradled me. Mom, being the determined woman that she is, laid on the floor because she refused to leave the room while he was there. She wanted me to know she wasn't going to take "no" for an answer and was so focused on "winning me over," as she always says.

She eventually did. The will and determination in her loving actions opened the door for me to accept the other women in my family. It was a very slow, tedious process, but it worked out better than I could've imagined. I spent my childhood and teenage years around very outspoken, strong-willed women, but I also grew up around strong, good-hearted boys and men, as well.

I'm my parents' only daughter through and through. I played with Power Ranger action figures instead of Barbie dolls, and listened to bands like Blink-182 and Linkin Park. It made me different, but I was never ashamed of those things; I embraced them—and still do. In fact, I still embrace a love for professional wrestling that my older brother instilled in me as a kid. However, there's more to my tomboy style than punk rock and pro wrestling.

Having been raised in a family of men who have shown me unconditional love in their own ways is something I'll always carry with me. It makes me want to be the best I can be —and maybe make a few people proud in the process. They never discouraged me from doing something just because I'm a female who happens to have a disability.

I have a father who holds strong to his actions and those of others, an uncle whose drive and creativity fuels me, two brothers who always have my back, and a grandfather who's now watching over me from above. I wouldn't ask for anything more, even if I could. My grandfather unfortunately never got to see my love of writing blossom into a career. That motivates me every day because he always told everyone he met, "My granddaughter is going to be the best writer in the world!"

If anything, growing up around men has given me a sense of pride. I've learned the value of hard work from listening to my grandfather's stories. I've listened to the way my dad opens the door after working long days at a local printing company. It's quiet observations like these that have helped me realize there will be times when I need to put my head down, get my hands dirty, and get things done. I'm also not afraid to put myself out there through my writing my story or my opinions.

All of these could have been bad for me. They weren't what anyone expected out of a little Korean girl, or the Korean woman I've grown to be. I welcome that, however. It gives me an opportunity to show people the real me.

It's not about being a woman. It's not about being adopted. It's not even about having a disability. It's instead about proving to myself that I am enough, and I can do anything.

Chapter 8

When Time Reveals the Ugly Truth

How to define your own independence.

Time is a precious, fleeting commodity. We want to bottle it and keep it forever. The problem is that every tick-tock of the clock is a piece of life's sand through the bend in the hourglass.

Time becomes the thing that reveals ugly truths about ourselves. Things we may not notice at first—or might not want to accept.

I realized time's trick when I had to go to physical therapy every day, had difficulty holding things in my hands, and couldn't even hold my head up for five minutes. I didn't have nearly as much independence as I would've liked to have, and knowing my situation wasn't likely to change fueled my desire to push forward.

I was around six or seven years old when everything in my orbit started to make sense. My disability was the sole reason why I didn't have complete freedom. It wasn't a matter of out-working everyone else around me to be comfortable. It wasn't even a situation where everything I did was met with questions like, *"Can she really do that on her own?"* or my least favorite of them all, *"Did you do that for her?"*

If anything, I needed to rise above other people's opinions about what I could or couldn't do. A shadow of doubt had been cast. I knew three things to be true up to this point:

1) I wasn't like everyone else;

2) I wasn't going to make excuses for myself; and, most importantly . . .

3) The world wasn't going to hand me whatever I wanted.

I wasn't quite sure what else to expect from the world at such a young age other than having confused, almost mesmerized stares drift in my direction. Even so, I felt certain that being spoon-fed was not on the list of things to anticipate. I did, however, have a budding passion for writing that started peeking through. It would eventually become one of the greatest assets of my life and provide the divine key to my independence.

That didn't mean I wasn't looking for ways to fill any voids I had in the meantime. Nor was I looking to impress anyone by trying to be as free and independent as my body would allow me to be. I simply wanted to experience the freedom of self-discovery. It was something that innately applied to my understanding of my diagnosis of cerebral palsy, so I wanted to see how I could apply it to other aspects of my life.

I also wanted a fair shot to mold myself into who and what I wanted to be. I didn't want to stay in the box society said I was supposed to be in. At the same time, however, I didn't want to be treated differently than anyone else. There was always a delicate balance as I got older. Ironically enough, my cerebral palsy slowly became the equalizer in all of this.

I needed to let go of my own insecurities about who or what I was. I needed to focus on the one thing that seemed to be rearing its head: my creativity. It had always been there in quiet, subtle ways—particularly in the fact that my disability made it difficult for me to speak. That, in turn, meant I wasn't being understood the way I wanted to be.

All the crayons, coloring books, glue and silly putty a kid could ever want kept my mind occupied for a while and even gave me a sense of freedom, but those vibes never seemed to be stronger or mightier than what I was feeling inside.

It got to the point where I'd had enough—enough of the doubt, the cold stares, the redundant questions. All of it. I knew then that I could no longer keep my love of creativity bottled up inside. It had become somewhat of a necessity at this point. So, I started writing. And writing.

And writing some more. It gave a genuine opportunity to break free from everything that was designed to hold me down. I loved how it made me feel, and I'd be stupid to let it go.

I didn't think of any of this as society's way of saying, *OK, it's time to grow up!* I saw it as an opportunity to mentally compensate for my lack of independence. If I couldn't be independent in my body, I was going to do everything in my power to be independent in my mind. Having done that through my writing and good old-fashioned hard work, it's ironic now to think I still don't have the independence I so yearn for. That is the truth—and when the truth becomes the headline of all of my stories, I know it's time to turn to a new page.

Chapter 9

Laugh Off the Wall

Wisdom of the best medicine.

We all need a break from our everyday routine sometimes, something to soften the heavy-handed punches life throws. We must stop and take a good look at ourselves when it seems like everything is too much too soon too often.

This wisdom has never steered me wrong. It's crucial to find a balance between reality and what's good about being alive. I just never thought these things would become the standard for how I choose to live my life.

I've always loved to laugh and find goodness in everything around me. My sense of humor is definitely spontaneous and a little off the wall. I've been known to burst into laughter at the smallest, most random things—like the pronunciation of an obscure word or the high pitched, chipmunk-like voice you get when you inhale helium from a balloon, among other things. There's just something about randomness that I love. And like the bond I share with the men in my family, I have no idea where it comes from.

It's an attribute that found a place in my life from an early age. The beginnings were there when I had to wear braces on my legs to help them grow properly when I was a kid. Or when a physical therapy session didn't go the way I envisioned it in my mind, despite giving it my all. Laughter was especially important when I woke up every morning and realized everything I had put my energy into on the day before were still feats that needed to be addressed and conquered again.

My appreciation for humor and laughter grew from there. I had all of these overwhelming factors from my cerebral palsy to contend with. I didn't know where to start or how to get the thought of always "getting things right" out of my head. It was like training for The Olympics because I was doing the same things every day, but missing a step in the process every time. When I had to have multiple surgeries on my legs, however, I thought the laughter would stop and the pain would start.

The pain did come, along with months of intense physical therapy for both of my legs. I had the surgeries done at Shriners Hospital for Children in Erie, Pennsylvania—where I was treated like a queen. The hospital is renowned for their expertise and care in helping young patients with disabilities. The staff took the time to work with my family to review my case and figure out what would be in my best interest before performing each surgery.

My physical therapists and doctors there stayed by my side every step of the way. The experience was probably the most fun I had as a kid. The staff had such a beautiful, creative approach to making me an essential part of my own healing process—whether I was cleaning up the mountain of toys from physical therapy or helping to change my bandages. The nurses even had activities and movies for patients every night, complete with popcorn and snacks. I brought home many crafts and "works of art" from those nights.

Everyone knew how to make things fun so kids would forget about their pain. It was a true gift, because I stayed at Shriners for weeks and months at a time. I was even known to hide in a few closets so that I did not have to face visiting clowns, which I feared. When I was finally healed enough to go home, I always fought it; I was having too much fun to leave! I'd fight back tears as I looked around to see other kids ready to go home, too. They would already be crying, begging to stay a little longer.

Those surgeries and long hospital stays were very painful, but they were also imperative to my physical and mental growth. I look back on those days with immense gratitude because they were some of my most difficult times. They were also some of my best because I learned how to laugh and have fun while dealing with my circumstances. I am also featured in a few articles and pictures in their anniversary book.

At the end of the day, that's what it's all about. I know I'm not going to wake up one day and all the baggage that comes with my disability will magically disappear. As great as that sounds, it's not my reality. I've learned to laugh because I feel like I'm wasting precious time if I don't. It's the only thing I have strength and energy to do some days, so I laugh until it hurts.

Laughter truly is the best medicine. So, however you decide to use it, make sure to do so wisely.

Chapter 10

How To Get the Goal When You Have To Go Back

You don't have to race to the finish line.

Mindsets change when going down those roads less traveled. You think you know where you're going but then end up in a completely different spot. The wind blows and things change even more.

I was quiet as a kid. I never wanted special treatment or to put the weight of my disability on anyone else's shoulders. I was always very independent in that sense and didn't want the little independence I had to be taken away. I was at the point where everything revolved around my wheelchair. I thought the cycle of those wheels turning in my head would never end, when I realized I needed to see for myself that I was wrong to think that way.

Going to school was my wake-up call. Most teachers weren't quite sure of how to react to me, which I expected. I had to show them I was worthy of being in "regular" classes. I had to prove why I didn't need to stay in the special inclusion class they had put me in. Granted, I wasn't forced to do this but

I wanted my teachers to look at me the way they looked at every other student. The weight of my responsibility suddenly had a new meaning.

A life-changing choice sparked this mindset. In second grade, my parents found out I wasn't doing my best in class. I had shut down during the day and refused to participate in activities or answer any questions. My mom became very curious and got permission to quietly sit in the back of class without me knowing she was there. What she saw immediately made her blood boil: me sitting at my desk, silently watching the world pass by.

She slowly walked to me after about five minutes and asked, "Are you doing your best?"

I shook my head no and before I could blink, we were in the car headed home. I was in tears at this point. I knew I was wrong—and nothing could smooth things over until I tried to explain.

Hours later, after the tears had dried, Mom asked me again if I was doing my best. I sat on the couch and cried until two simple words came out of my mouth: "No challenge."

I was confronted by my teacher the very next day. Why was I so quiet and dismissive in class? At that moment, the stage was set for everything I'd do from that point on:

"Do you want to stay in the inclusion class for half a day, or repeat second grade and be mainstreamed into regular classes?"

I chose the latter without hesitation not thinking about the tremendous impact it would end up having on my life. Or that it might help others see me as something more than the girl in a wheelchair. I wanted to prove to myself there was something beyond my disability—a wall I didn't have to bust through to be comfortable with myself.

The decision to repeat the second grade was a huge step in that process. It was my decision, and it was the best one I would ever make. But just when I thought I was on a somewhat steady path, life threw a major curveball my way.

In elementary school—about fourth grade—I had a second surgery on my legs and had to be homeschooled during my recovery. I had a double cast, one on each leg, with a big bar between that made it extremely difficult to move or do anything. I had to get comfortable with pain and not going to school.

I said goodbye to the friends I'd made and assured them I'd be back. My teacher was willing to come to our house every day to go over what he'd taught in class, and it turned out to be one of the best things for me.

He would stay until he had gone over everything and gave me the materials to complete the work I had missed. That kind of support is always welcome. He knew I'd had major surgery and went out of his way to help lighten my load.

My teacher doing all of this on his own time made it even more meaningful. It wasn't the first encounter I would have with a true teacher. In fact, this set the stage for the enriching exchanges I had with teachers over the years. Major life exchanges are always easier said than done, especially when the weight is all on your own shoulders because others rarely know how capable we are.

At the end of the day, I learned it truly takes a village to raise a child. Many teachers were the cornerstones of my village—and still are. I'm beyond grateful to have such bright, intelligent minds willing to guide my choices as a writer and a human being.

These teachers have shown me it doesn't matter how you start. It's how you finish that counts—and I'm not even close to my finishing line.

My wheels are still rolling---forward or backward---but they don't define me or my abilities; only my goals---my finishing lines---do. So, what are you willing to do to get to your goal, what do you want at the end of your finishing line?

Chapter 11

When Frustration Occurs Again and Again

How to make sense of it all.

The world is full of pitfalls and false truths. They can lead us to places we don't want to go or bring us back to the very spot we spend so much time and effort trying to get away from. The tiny voices in our head may tell us that those places aren't as bad as we remember, and invite us back in.

That's the moment when we question ourselves and quietly ask, "Why did I allow myself to fall into this trap again?" Then we wonder where we might have taken a wrong turn. That was me at ten or eleven years old.

All of the frustrations I had about not being able to do certain things on my own started to resurface. All the emotions that were attached to them came rushing back, as well. These things were always there and I thought I had conquered them, but I was wrong. The fact that I didn't like when things changed wasn't making for an easy transition into being a disabled kid with not one but two bum legs. Not only that, but I also had to keep up with my schoolwork while I was recovering from my surgery.

I had to make some sense of my circumstances on top of fighting bouts of radiating pain. I had what felt like 100-pound weights on my legs due to the double cast that I had on for months. That also led to countless hours of physical therapy, which were excruciatingly painful some days. It just seemed like the weight of having cerebral palsy was amplified by having surgery to the point where it put me in a very uncomfortable position. I already felt like a burden by default, and I was striking out even more.

Admittedly, I was frustrated.

That's saying a lot because I don't get frustrated easily. This, however, pushed me to what I thought was my breaking point. I didn't know whether to laugh, cry or have a nervous breakdown. It was like being trapped in my own body, more so than before. I was OK when I only had my disability to deal with. It somehow made me feel strong because I had finally figured out how to overcome that part of my life.

I still had fears and doubts about it, but I knew I could rise above them. They were nothing new. Now, however, there were these other painfully heavy obstacles being thrown into the mix. My only saving grace was knowing that both of my surgeries were over, and they were going to help me in the long run.

That's not to say I still didn't feel angry or overwhelmed by my situation. I knew I had to have surgery. Yet, I was completely unprepared for the waves of emotion it would bring. This was something I didn't want to put on anyone else's shoulders any more than I had to. It would have been wrong of me to put that pressure on my family, so I did the only thing I knew how to do: put my head down and push through the pain.

In hindsight, it wasn't the smartest thing I've ever done. My determination to get through this taught me a lot about developing thicker skin, but it also made it harder for me to ask for help. It was harder, still, to deny that I needed help. I wasn't trying to be cocky or selfish; I just wanted to grow up in my own way, and my own pain gave me that opportunity.

The one thing I relied on then is still true for me now: my ability to focus on a single task until it is finished. That also allows me to be less afraid of my daily shortcomings and to be OK with the fact that they're always going to be there. If anything, having surgery reminded me of that.

I don't think I will ever be fine with not being able to do simple, everyday things on my own. It's not anything I hold against my family, society, or even myself. It's a matter of knowing that even when my back is always against the wall in some way, I fight my way out.

It's always important to remember why you do what you do, and why you stick with it. I found my reasons for fighting through frustration. What are yours?

Chapter 12

How To Use What You Have

Some of us come with a lot of baggage.

Every day is a new day. It's an opportunity to step up and go a little further than the day before. A chance to embrace things that might have been there for the taking all along, but something gets in the way.

We learn a lot about ourselves when we try to move whatever that thing may be. We might have some help or we might not. When we have help, it's easier to see what needs to be done. And how to do it. When help isn't within reach, however, we sometimes realize the mountain that needs to be moved is one that we must move on our own.

I came to a somewhat different conclusion as I got older. I had help around me. I always have, and I'm extremely grateful for it. The difference is that I've never liked to abuse the fact that it's always there, which I could easily do. However, I try to figure out when I need the most help before asking for it. It's something that I don't take lightly because my need for assistance is apparent – and it always will be.

Looking back, knowing I had all that extra baggage when I was younger makes me feel like I could've somehow done more for myself. Or at least not have had to be so reliant during that time. I had help outside of my family, too.

There was a point where I even asked myself, *Are people helping me because they genuinely want to, or are they doing it because it's what's expected when they see someone like me? Or is it a little bit of both?*

That was also when I told myself I needed to start carrying my own weight. I wanted to try to do more for myself. Help myself. But how? I couldn't make money, drive a car, cook or do laundry. That was the extent of what I thought encompassed an adult's world. It was everything I heard my parents tell my older brother, so I thought it applied to me as well.

I remembered the communication board I had in second grade, and the impact it had on my life. It was the very first piece of technology that I learned to use. It certainly wouldn't be the last, but the way it made me feel stayed with me. I wanted that feeling of freedom and responsibility again. So, I asked my parents for the one thing I thought could fill that void – a cell phone.

"Why do you need a phone?" they asked.

"Well, it could be useful…" I said.

I wasn't trying to make a big deal out of it. I wasn't trying to be a cool kid or bribe my parents into buying me my first phone, either. I genuinely thought it would be a wise investment for me at the time. Not only that, but the notion that I could still get help if it wasn't nearby eased my mind. On that note, my parents agreed to let me get a phone. It would end up being a measure of safety because my family was always on the go. They still are.

As an adult now, I appreciate the fact I can reach my family wherever they may be. I also appreciate that I've learned to use and view technology as a legitimately useful tool to help me live my life the way I want to live it, rather than making it convenient and easy. I respect the fact that most people use technology because of its convenience and ease. That's what it's made for. I just hope that others respect the fact that technology was – and still is, my lifeline in many ways.

However, it's hard to shed some of that weight when I know it's still going to be there tomorrow – just in a different form. It was even harder to not feel that way when I was a kid. I at least have something to help lift that heaviness off my shoulders, and I couldn't be more grateful.

I come with a lot of baggage. I didn't want to lose sight of that when I was younger — and I definitely don't want to let it slip my mind now. Learning how to use technology — whether it's my computer, cell phone or my motorized wheelchair, has. It's one of the few ways I can be self-reliant without feeling like I'm bothering anyone else.

Use what you have. That's one of the most important things I've learned. It might not be given to you or passed down from another generation. You may have to find it yourself. And when you do find it, don't waste it.

Chapter 13

The Measure of Maturity

When you fight for your future with thought.

Some people say life is meant to be lived and we should keep our eyes open and be present in every moment. Others say life just happens and we need to take whatever comes our way.

These two schools of thought can mold and shape everything around us. They're powerful on their own without any bells or whistles. Although they may be contested at times, our thoughts can't be taken away from us.

They're ours. We own them, but something has to happen to make us think the way that we do.

The notion that things just happen without rhyme or reason has never set well with me. Nor has the idea that the things that do happen don't leave a lasting impact on you or someone else around you. That way of thinking didn't help me or mark a path of maturity for me. At the time, I didn't realize how true this was. Nor how important it would become. It didn't make me think any less of myself, either. In fact, it did the opposite.

It motivated me.

It made me realize I didn't need a typical rite of passage to signify that I was mature. I slowly came to the conclusion that I could rely on my thought process to measure my own maturity. My thoughts had never been childish up until this point because they always had to be doing something for me – whether they acted as my moral compass when I was in pain, or guided a choice I'd made when I was a kid.

I eventually came to another conclusion. The reason I was so headstrong wasn't so much because I learned the ways of the world at a young age. It was rather because I had to fight to get to where I was – fight to reach a point in my life where it was plausible to think about my future. And to even have a future beyond the realm of my cerebral palsy. So now, here I was. 12 or 13 years old, with nothing but my thoughts and budding ambitions to carry me.

I hadn't done anything big with my passion for writing yet. I also didn't have the privilege of eventually receiving many of the things most kids my age dreamed of getting: a car, keys or a driver's license – among other rites of passage. That hope was dashed before I even knew how I truly felt about it. All I had was the cell phone that I convinced my parents to let me buy, which I treasured.

My phone gave me a genuine sense of independence and responsibility. It was almost equal to the feeling that my first motorized wheelchair gave me – as well as the other pieces of technology I'd learned to use over the years. The emotion they evoked in my soul was immeasurable, but I felt I had nothing else to show for myself.

That started to get under my skin. I was waiting for something to happen. Something that could let me know I was truly growing up. I had already been through enough to know that a negative mindset wasn't going to get me anywhere. And it didn't.

I wasn't trying to be something I wasn't. I was simply trying to get through this extremely awkward stage in my life. It was very clear that my path to maturity wasn't going to be lined with fancy things. I accepted that, but I struggled to fill a void that I couldn't explain or describe.

I tried being angry. I tried being bitter and taking my frustrations out on people who didn't deserve to be yelled at or ridiculed. Or had nothing to do with my circumstances. None of my tactics were working, so I tapped back into what I've always known: the power of determination. That, along with a slight change in attitude, brought me to a better place. It was a place where I didn't have to be angry or bitter. Nor did I want to be.

I could just accept the fact that things were different for me, even the smallest things. I remind myself that if I can't physically be as strong and poised as I'd like to be, my thoughts are stronger. They're always there to fill that empty space and I am grateful for that.

If the mind is considered a great and useful tool, I'd like to think I've used mine well. It's yet another gift that shouldn't be wasted. As with any gift that's found, not given.

Chapter 14

Age Has a Funny Way of Changing Your Life

Growing older changes the way we see, hear and feel.

Age might even change how we think, but the key is to not lose sight of what brought us to where we are in the first place.

Our journey to get where we want to be might force us to leave many things behind. Our means of getting there may not be conventional or expected. We're sometimes met with raised eyebrows and cringed faces when we decide to go against the grain and follow an unexplored path. As I'd find out, however, the road that's less traveled is often the one with the greatest reward.

My reward didn't come as quickly as one might think. I didn't expect it to, because my path had been far from normal so far. I had a sneaking feeling it was going to stay that way for a long time, if not for the rest of my life. I couldn't have asked anyone else to travel this path. It wouldn't have been fair because that responsibility wasn't theirs. It was mine – and I knew it.

Not only that, but I knew staying on the path I'd been on was going to be much easier said than done. Many things up until this point were. I was now getting ready to "graduate" from elementary school and start junior high. I looked at it as a new chapter in my life, one in which I could possibly begin building my world – or at least parts of it – around something other than my disability. More than anything, however, I thought this was a real chance to gain more independence.

It was painfully obvious by now that I was never going to get away from making cerebral palsy the centerpiece of my existence. I couldn't simply cross it off my list of things that demanded my attention. Everyone around me knew that and respected it for the most part. I also understood the fact that technology had impacted my life in a very personal, intimate way. It wasn't just there for ease and aesthetics.

That quickly became one of the most important things I wanted other people to understand as well. I was willing to do whatever it took to get that point across. More than that, however, I still had so much to prove to myself and others. Little did I know, I'd have an opportunity to do just that by the end of sixth grade.

My class was asked to write book reports about influential figures in American history. I chose Harriet Tubman and, like my classmates, I checked out books from the school library and did my own research. I quietly started typing my paper on my communication board, hoping I would get a solid paragraph or two written before the school day was over.

It didn't happen, even though I worked diligently.

I took my paper home to finish it that night and transfer it to my parents' computer to print out. Most of my teachers were aware that this would be a regular occurrence because it took me longer to complete my assignments.

Fast forward to around 11 p.m. I could barely keep my eyes open as I cringed while typing the very last line of my paper. I knew more about Tubman than I ever thought I'd know, but I was OK with that because I was finally finished with this assignment. I proudly read it over before taking it to school the next day.

When I handed it in, however, my teacher looked very confused. She was almost in disbelief. So much so that she gave it back to me after a few minutes. There were no pen marks on it. No comments.

"Erin, you didn't write this yourself," my teacher said with a disgusted scowl on her face.

"Yes, I did," I explained. "I finished it at home last night on the computer, without any help."

"First of all, this is too well-written to be yours…"

I could tell from there that this exchange wasn't going very far. No amount of convincing was going to change my teacher's mind. While I didn't have proof that I wrote the paper on my own, she knew I didn't finish it in class the day before. She also knew that I had to take it home to do the rest.

This turned into a 20-minute debacle, which resulted in me having to do a second research paper. I was hurt, angry and crying at this point. I was confused for a few minutes, but I realized this was yet another test of my determination. It did, however, bring back a flood of unpleasant memories.

My personal care aide, who helped me in class, watched this entire scene unfold and came to my defense. She advised me to write another paper, even though both my parents and I fought against it. I was angry at the fact the fact my teacher didn't trust me by my own merit. Writing that second paper wasn't the problem. In fact, I worked on it for about a week and turned it in.

It had the same quality as the first one. The same care and attention to detail. My teacher was completely silent when she saw this. I wasn't sure if she didn't know what to say, or just didn't want to honestly acknowledge what had happened. Either way, I felt at ease knowing I kept up my end of this.

I didn't get an apology from her until many years later.

Maybe my teacher wanted to show me tough love. Maybe she wanted to make an example out of me and my writing. I don't know, but whatever her reasoning was, it worked.

I'm a better person because of it. This wouldn't be the last time I faced doubt, however.

It goes to show that people will never know who you truly are unless you show them. They might not believe it at first, but that's when you give it all you've got. And if you give enough of yourself, a few eyes are bound to be opened.

Chapter 15

Dangerous, Delicate Power

If you want power and control, are you also willing to earn it?

Power is a dangerous, yet delicate thing. It can overcome us, and make us feel like we're on top of the world. It can give us access to things we may never have dreamed.

It's easy to think the world is ours for the taking when power is given. It can poison our bodies and minds. When power is earned or awarded, however, we can make our own way, dream our own dreams and maybe even learn to use what we have to make something worthwhile. Or at least, dream bigger.

That's one thing I've always tried to do, regardless of the many things I don't have power or control of in my own life. It has always been important for me to work with the things I do have, rather than wish for what I don't. That can range from my ability to feed myself to the way I think on any given day. I embrace those little things more than I readily admit because they empower me. I try to balance that empowerment with the fact that the world isn't tailor-made to accommodate my disability. Nor the emotions that are attached to it.

I learned very quickly the world doesn't come pre-packaged. It's not an object that you can take out of a box and expect it to be perfect. There's some assembly required, and I'm willing to build until I can't build anymore. My cerebral palsy is a constant reminder that I need to mold my surroundings in a way that suits my needs. Most importantly, I need to do so mindfully and realistically.

I've applied this mindset to every aspect of my life and it has benefited me. It even helped me through my transition when I started junior high. I was already a curious, awkward kid. Now, I was a curious, awkward kid in an equally strange position. But that was all about to change.

I was still in grade school when I was preparing to receive my first motorized wheelchair. My parents felt I was responsible enough to handle a new set of wheels, and I was ready to show them they were right. I didn't mind I had to wait until I was a little older. Nor that I had to go to driving school – and pass – before everything was official. I was just excited to have a real chance to gain a little bit more independence.

I was also very nervous because I had never even sat in a motorized wheelchair before – let alone driven one. All I remember having was a hot pink wheelchair with rickety wheels and an oversized seat. It was the talk of my neighborhood when I was younger.. Now, however, here I was – sitting in class on a somewhat warm day, waiting for the final bell to ring. The hot, sticky mesh-like fabric on the cushion of my small manual chair was sticking to the back of my legs. That was usually enough for me to count the seconds until the bell rang every day. On this particular day, however, there was an extra boost of anxiousness.

The bell finally rang after a few long minutes. The local school van picked me up and drove me home. My parents transferred me to their car and we were off to the wheelchair clinic. We soon entered a large room with plenty of space to drive around. There were orange cones scattered across the floor and tape marked off different areas. My eyes were fixed on the sleek wheelchair parked nearby, which I hoped to call my own. Or at least one like it.

A gentleman walk in a few minutes later, smiled and asked, "Are you ready to give this thing a spin?"

"Yes!" I eagerly replied.

With that, I got in the chair and slowly navigated my way around the course. I tried not to let anyone see how shaky I was. I didn't know if I'd get another opportunity like this, so I blocked everything else out and just drove. When I looked back to see if I had knocked anything over about two hours later, my eyes filled up with hot tears.

All the cones were still standing. The tape on the floor wasn't folded or bent – and to my surprise, I could drive in a straight line. Everything was still in its place. The gentleman who was monitoring me and giving me directions shot me a wink of approval.

I left driving school feeling incredibly rewarded, even though I had to wait another few weeks until I got my own chair after customizing and ordering it. I went to school with newfound self-respect. I not only passed the latest test in life, but I also gained the power I always thought was missing.

That motorized chair would be the first of many I'd eventually call my own. I realize now that having this type of chair is perhaps the greatest power I will ever have because it isn't about independence and getting what I want. It's about what I choose to do with the things my chair gives me that I didn't have before.

We all want power over our own lives. We all want to have some sort of control. But are you willing to earn it? Or let someone hand it to you?

Chapter 16

How To Develop a Quiet Respect

Not everyone sees what you see; can you help them?

Are the best things in life worth waiting for? If we wait for the right moment, will everything fall into place? Should we seize the opportunities we are given?

Some might say it's redundant to wait for an opportunity when we can create it ourselves. If we're willing to take risks, we might give other people a reason to believe in something. The same thing could happen if we're willing to be vulnerable. The rewards that come from that alone, however, can make us richer than any millionaire.

My cerebral palsy makes me vulnerable by default. There's no denying that, nor is there a clever way of getting around it. It's a cold, hard fact of my existence – one that has never been easy to confront. However, I try to remember that having a disability is often a double-edged sword. It may tear me apart some days, but it ultimately makes me stronger because the struggle will always be there. I work on overcoming it every day.

I look at certain things – like my phone or my wheelchair – to remind myself that every day doesn't have to be a struggle. I have technology to thank for that. Every device I use has a specific role in my life, and I've learned each of their tricks to near perfection. That's not to say the very things I rely on are never the root of a bad day, though. They indeed are. It's yet another reminder of why I can't refuse help – whether it's offered to me or not.

As I would find out, however, the way in which certain devices are used can also serve as a measure of respect. My need for technology has followed me wherever I go. It's very apparent in almost everything I do. Being introduced to technology in the manner I was – and at the pace in which I was thrown into that world – taught me many valuable lessons about humility and being humble in the most personally difficult times.

They weren't lessons I necessarily wanted to learn at an early age. They were more bullet points on the long list of things I had to learn to accept – and having a motorized wheelchair helped with that process. In truth, I wanted to be hanging out with friends or doing anything other than learning how to use technology. But I understood the bells and whistles that accompanied me weren't for show. I wanted other people to see as well.

I'd been using a motorized chair for many years by the time I got to junior high school. I also had a specially-programmed laptop computer, which I found much easier to use than the communication board I had used. I never did acquire the speed that comes with being a proficient typist, but I have accuracy and efficiency. That was all I needed.

Everyone in school slowly noticed how carefully and meticulously I typed: with my right hand, delicately pressing one key at a time with my index finger. It's the same way I still type to this day. When I'd look up from my computer screen, eyebrows would raise and a few doubts might have even been erased.

My classmates and teachers also started watching how easily I could parallel park my chair right next to my assigned seat in class. They started complimenting me on my driving skills and even knew when I was coming down the hallways, by listening for the echoing click of my motor. As time went on, I could feel a shift in the way I was treated. There was also a change in the way I was being perceived.

All of this felt strange at first, but I welcomed it. I began to feel like maybe – just maybe – my cerebral palsy wasn't the center of attention anymore. I thought, *Maybe people are finally seeing what I've been trying to show them for all these years!*

The little things I was doing weren't things I particularly wanted to highlight about myself. Nor were these things I thought anyone would pick up on. They were a part of my everyday life, but people began to pay attention to how and why I did what I did. Little did I know, however, a kind of quiet respect would carry over into other aspects of my life.

Sometimes people don't see what you see. They may need a little more help, or they might even need you to guide the way. Will you be up for that challenge?

Chapter 17

Mutual Respect Showdown

How to keep a tight grip on confidence.

When something good comes into our lives, we tend to hold onto it a little tighter. We keep it close to our hearts and learn everything we can from it. We might not want it to end, but sometimes we don't have a choice.

In the process of coming to terms with that, however, we can often become comfortable. Too comfortable, perhaps to the point where we forget that things like peace of mind and calmness aren't always a given.

We have to let go of automatic comfort at some point, whether it's brought into our lives by a certain person, place or thing. It's not always easy like flipping a switch or cracking a smile. It might not even come in the form of a harsh goodbye or a difficult lesson that needed to be learned.

It might just simply be a mutual show of respect between two people. That's exactly what it was for me as I got older and realized that comfort – at least my own – had to be earned just like everything else in my life. I got my chance when I came face-to-face with one of my tenth-grade teachers, who completely changed my perspective of what a teacher was supposed to be.

With that came a different view of the way a teacher carried themselves and conducted business in the classroom. It was something I had never encountered in all the years that I'd been going to school. Not only that, but I would soon gain the tools I needed to truly move on to bigger and better things in life.

Technology helped me do that in a big way, but I knew the rest was up to me. And me alone. I had gotten through junior high with a growing confidence that people saw there was more to me than just my cerebral palsy, having written for my school newspapers every year. It was a feeling that I wasn't completely familiar with because of past experiences. Now it was time to see how far it would take me as I entered high school.

It was a breezy end-of-summer day in 2001, about forty-eight hours before the start of my sophomore year I was running through my schedule and meeting my teachers for the first time, with my mom by my side. The bleach-blonde sun brightened and faded through a high window, spilling its light down a corridor of classrooms.

The clickity-click of the motor in my wheelchair echoed through thick, empty walls. I passed at least two-dozen rooms, doors shut with lights on, before stopping at the last room at the end of the hall – room 329, biology.

The door was open. My eyes immediately traced the circular pattern in the wood, and I prayed it wouldn't trace back to the days when I was just "a girl in a wheelchair". I drove a few feet further to see a lumberjack-like silhouette of gentle quietness, hunched over at the desk in the front of the room with a pen in hand.

"Hi there. Are you Erin?" the tall, burly man with a clean-cut goatee asked, as he calmly put the pen down and stood up. His shadow filled the doorframe when he walked into the hallway. I waited for it to lag behind, but it spilled onto the marbled linoleum floor outside his classroom. I felt like I was looking up at The Eiffel Tower.

He extended a handshake right away. My fingers were sprawled like limbs on a naked body.

I nodded a decisive "yes" to his question, but my mind was fishing for proof that my chair didn't define who I was.

"I'm Mr. DeAntonio. Mr. D. for short," he said without a glance at my mom. "I heard you coming down the hall. Are you a good student?"

"Well, I try." My head flew off its hinges again. I couldn't put my finger on it, but there was something welcoming about the diplomatic tone of his voice.

"It takes her longer to finish her assignments, and she'll need somebody to take her notes," my mom chimed in.

She didn't say much during the hour-and-a-half we spent in that hallway as she took in the scene that was unfolding in front of her.

"We can work with that," Mr. D. calmly replied. "No worries. If we run into any problems in class, I expect Erin to help me out. I can already tell she's a smart cookie!"

This was it. This was the kind of treatment I'd been waiting so long for. It was exactly what I had been asking people to do. The fact this was coming from someone who would simultaneously shape me as a human being, was even more impressive. All of this was done very quietly, but it was also very obvious at the same time. Mr. D. demanded respect, and he expected the same from his students.

He wasn't trying to pull the wool over my eyes. He wasn't trying to convince me that he was radically different than any teacher I'd ever had up to this point, either. He had a very simple, straight-forward approach to teaching, which carried over into the way he treated others. I knew he expected the same from me as his other students, and he was encouraging in helping to find ways for me to do things in class, on my own.

I felt like I was on my way to finding my place in the world, but I wouldn't have to do it alone. Mr. D. was – and still is – one of the many people in my life who saw something special in me before I knew what to do with it.

It had nothing to do with my cerebral palsy. He made a remark that I will remember forever: "All students have a problem, some you can see, others you don't."

Good things may come and go. They might even be disguised as a big, towering mountain you have to climb, but don't loosen your grip. You might miss out on something great.

Chapter 18

Trust Your Gut

Ideas connect us to everything.

Ideas are the gateway to bigger ambitions and even bigger dreams. Most importantly, ideas can be the start of something great. Sometimes all we need is a little push. Or a little reminder of why we do what we do.

Other times, however, it takes more than that. Sometimes it's a matter of what we do when our backs are against the wall. It's about what we choose to do when no one is looking – or not expecting us to do anything at all.

I had an idea of finally doing something with my passion for writing – or explore it, at the very least. It had always been there, ready to burst out like a jack-in-a-box while I was busy dealing with everyday life. But it was my everyday routine – my wheelchair driving, button-pushing routine I had learned to call life. I didn't think it was boring, but it was something to start with.

It was something I built with my own two hands. I was happy about that, probably the happiest I'd been in a long time. At this point, I had a fairly good sense of how words fit together on a page. My three years of serving as a staff writer for the school newspaper in junior high was the only formal introduction to writing that I had up until that point.

Granted, there was an expected wave of doubt and shock that came over the adviser's face when I first rolled into the room. At the time, being a writer for the newspaper was actually a class you could get credit for. I signed up for the class, so the adviser knew I was coming. I don't think she expected me to be in a wheelchair, though. When I turned in a draft of my first story a few weeks later, however, the vibes were completely different. The shock was still there, but a lot of the doubt had melted away.

I knew I had broken through a very high glass ceiling at that moment. If I wanted to do the same in high school, it would undoubtedly be a process. I would have to prove myself, which had become second nature to me. I developed a quiet confidence in my ability to write as a result of having to prove myself countless times over the years. I also now had solid reassurance that people were looking beyond my cerebral palsy. The first-hand experience I gained from writing in junior high, along with my own personal need to express myself, was my fuel to try to write as much as my teachers would allow me to. And prove my worth to an entirely new group of people.

If I made it on the staff of my high school newspaper, I'd be one step closer to perhaps gaining even more confidence. If I didn't make it, however, I wanted to learn as much as I could about the craft of writing. I wanted to catch lightning in a bottle either way. Writing proved to be an extremely important – almost vital – part of my existence. I certainly wasn't going to be complacent about the possibility of doing it more often, on whatever scale I could.

Not wanting to pass up an opportunity that came my way, I secretly wanted to earn a spot on my high school newspaper's staff. I didn't want it to be handed to me just because someone felt pity for me like, *Aww, she wants to write. What a nice thought!* No. I wanted to show people that I *could* write, and my willingness to make an impression wasn't some outlandish impulse.

This was so much more. I wanted to make a good impression, but I also felt like I had a responsibility. Writing was the first thing, other than my disability, that gave me a sense of purpose. It gave me another big reason to prove myself and my worth. I hoped this all would eventually become apparent to others if nothing else. All I needed was a small opening – an inch, two inches or however much space someone was willing to give me.

I took this mindset into my sophomore year of high school, all the way to the adviser of the school newspaper. I politely waited for the look of shock on his face to go away before asking, "Would you mind if I give this a shot?"

There was a long pause. Then silence. I could tell he was doubtful by the shaky tone of his voice.

"Well," he said. "What experience [with writing] do you have?"

My mind was searching for a subtle way to say I didn't have any formal experience. I waited a few more minutes to tell him that I'd been referred by the adviser of my junior high newspaper, to continue to write for the high school's paper.

Again, it was a matter of signing up for the class. I just didn't want my potential adviser and teacher to be surprised this time around.

There was another pause – shorter than the one before. I waited to see if that was good or bad.

More silence…

"Welcome aboard!"

With that reply, I made it a point to work harder than I ever had in my life. I didn't have a literary agent, nor did I have a way into the writing industry. One thing was for sure, however. I was going to make sure that this adviser – or anyone else who I'd possibly write for – didn't regret their decision to take a chance on me.

This certainly wasn't the end of the ride, but I was going to enjoy it. I just remembered typing random things out on my computer. I had fond memories of my now outdated communication board, and how long it took to "graduate" from using one device to the next. What a crazy journey – one that's just getting started!

Trust your gut. It may sound like simple, almost cheesy rhetoric. As I found out, it's not. It's the key to truly living a fulfilled life.

Chapter 19

Mindsets Change To Rise Above the Negative

The ability to look at something from someone else's point of view without judgment is a precious gift.

This gift doesn't come in wrapping paper. Nor is it topped with a shiny bow. It's a gift that's only given when it is earned.

The same can be said about the ability to see something good in things that aren't always viewed as positive. The notion that we may be going through the same situation as someone else is common. The way in which we find a way out of that situation, however, is what makes us who we are. Some might even say it sets us apart from the other person, along with everyone else.

I've always tried to find the silver lining in having cerebral palsy because I'd be letting myself down every single day if I didn't. There's a certain amount of pride in knowing I'm not the only person in the world with a disability – something I've accepted as unique. Yet, I don't look at it as being a part of a special club or group that should be treated differently than any other group or demographic.

I've also tried my best to put myself in the shoes of someone on the outside looking in, who might not understand the daily complexities of my circumstances. Or might think that being in a wheelchair is anything less than what it actually is for me: a constant, quiet effort to make things work in a somewhat smooth and independent manner. As I was making my way through high school, however, I began to notice something that I'd never seen or experienced before.

I was looking at my cerebral palsy as a positive thing, but not everyone around me shared the same sentiment. I encountered people who thought my circumstances were a hindrance and a bad omen of sorts. I didn't know what to think at first, because I was so used to hearing things like, "Aww, poor baby!" and "You can't do this or that!" They were hurtful comments that I learned to brush off. On the other hand, they were never twisted and turned until my disability sounded like I would be cursed for the rest of my life.

I didn't mind the fact that others had different viewpoints about my circumstances. It was natural, just like the way people have their own opinions about anything else in this world. I welcomed those opinions because I was genuinely interested in what people had to say. Some would even comment on how much weight my disability put on my shoulders, and how difficult it must be to overcome it. I didn't argue with those individuals or any of the points they were making, because they were absolutely true.

However, the comments slowly turned into things like, "Oh, I wish I had one of those [wheelchairs]. It must be so much fun driving around in it!" or "You have it so easy, being in that chair!" At this point, I didn't know whether to laugh or cry as a result of the misguided envy that was pouring out of these comments.

It's not that they weren't heartfelt. It wasn't even that this was coming from little kids who didn't know any better, or people who didn't have a disability. This came from everyone, from my peers to complete strangers who were young, old and seemingly every age in between. I wanted to be angry. I wanted to scream, *Why would anyone want anything I have, let alone think it's fun?* I told myself that the people who were saying most of these things didn't know the whole story. And might never know the whole story.

They were simply making observations based on what they saw, which was me driving around in my motorized wheelchair – looking like everything was OK. What they didn't know, however, was that it had taken me many years to feel comfortable with my cerebral palsy. Not only that, but those individuals were miles ahead of me while I was still trying to cross the starting line. It took me that long to get to where I was going or to do whatever I was trying to do – and it still does.

This happened frequently enough that I started to think people wanted to believe that the hand I'd been dealt was indeed a hindrance. I also started asking myself, *Are they trying to convince themselves? Or me?* Maybe that was their way of being polite when they didn't know how to approach me. Maybe they had never seen someone in a wheelchair before, who's as alert and cognitive as I'm fortunate enough to be.

I may never know the real reason, but I didn't need any convincing that my life was anything less than what I made it out to be instead of what everyone thought it was. If I convinced myself that my disability was a bad thing, that's what it was going to be. By the same token, it was only going to be a hindrance if I let it get in my way.

People's mindsets slowly started to change once they saw that my circumstances were what built me up rather than tore me down. Their perception changed to the point where I no longer have to deal with the majority of the things I did when I was younger. I can't attribute that to just one thing, but I've found an abundance of motivation in unlikely places. Even so, I still see some of that misled glorification coming through at times.

It goes to show that you shouldn't listen to all the noise around you. Sometimes you need to take it with a grain of salt. It doesn't mean you don't hear what people say. It just means you're strong enough to rise above negativity.

Chapter 20

Life Throws Curveballs When We Least Expect It

Sometimes they're small and somewhat avoidable. Other times, however, they're so big that we can't ignore them.

We might not even be able to put some curveballs to the side because we don't see them coming. There may be times when we have to immediately deal with whatever is thrown at us, even though the effects might stay with us. There might even be a time when we're pulled in the opposite direction of where we're going. Either something happens that changes our course or someone tries to sway our decisions.

That's the very moment when we have to pause, step back and find a bigger picture we're not seeing at a given moment. We also have to decide if we like the picture being painted – and how we can make changes without tarnishing what's already there.

My last two years of high school taught me the most difficult curveballs are the ones you can't completely get away from. It would be easy, almost expected, for me to say my disability had been somewhat of a setback during this time. It would be even easier to say it was a setback all along, but that wouldn't be a genuine truth.

There were other things in my life bigger than my disability: making and losing friends, spending time with my loved ones and figuring out what my next step was as it related to my writing.

I was in my junior year, preparing to make some big decisions about the year ahead. My mind was set on going to college and pursuing a major that involved writing. So, I carefully scheduled my classes for my senior year with that in mind. I didn't want there to be any doubt or suspicion I didn't meet the requirements needed to graduate.

I had come too far for something like that to happen, and I was going to do everything in my power to make sure it didn't. I wanted to do things the right way because I knew everything I did now mattered more than ever.

I was also aware my family was supportive of my ambition to go to college, even though I wouldn't be the first to do so. My grandparents wore their pride on their sleeve when it came to their grandchildren. There was an added layer of motivation to not only go to college, but to also do the best I possibly could.

I was looking forward to spending the summer with my family, with my intentions clear and my junior year of high school now coming to a close. I got my wish, but my world completely changed as things began to thaw out from the cold, hard winter that followed.

The air was still crisp when I came home from school on March 28, 2003. It was one year before I was set to graduate. My dad, who had an unusual look on his face, greeted me as I got off the van that drove me to school every morning. I couldn't quite figure out why he had such a solemn look, or what it meant. I motored my way off of the push-button lift attached to the van until my wheels touched the gravel in our driveway.

I was a bit confused as to why my mom wasn't home too, because she always walked over the bridge on our property to come get me after school. I wanted to say something, but I didn't know what would be appropriate in this moment.

"Hey toots!", my dad said. "How was school?"

"Good…" I waited a few minutes before asking, "Where's Mom?"

"She had to take care of something with Nana. They'll be back."

About an hour later, my mom's van pulled into the driveway. I heard doors open and then a long, drawn-out pause. My mom slowly walked into the house with her mother, Nana, in tow. They could barely hold back tears as they came into my room.

"Erin," Mom squeaked out through her burst of emotion. "I have to tell you something…"

She grabbed my hand and squeezed tightly before telling me my grandfather, "Honey," as I called him, had passed away early that morning, after suffering a heart attack. I immediately became angry and lost complete control. I balled up my first and hit the wall, but my tiny hand had no force behind it.

I didn't want to believe it. I refused to believe it, because my grandfather had a history of heart attacks and cardiovascular issues due to severe diabetes. He made it through all of that and then some. Not only that, but he taught me so much about what it means to live and love fiercely. There was no way *this* heart attack was the one that took him away from us.

The more I denied what I had just heard, the tighter my mom held me. She knew this would break me because this would be the first of three grandparents I'd lose. And it happened to be the one I was closest to. As Mom tried to calm me down, other family members held my hand and joined in our huddle. My nana wiped away her own tears, leaned in and said, "It's true, Erin."

My grandfather's death marked the beginning of a new, personal struggle – one I still deal with today. It also made me work harder and prepared me for some of the worst times in my life. I take those lessons with me wherever I go and try to pay it forward every day.

Whatever your wealth is, share it. Don't hide it. It may not seem like much to you, but it could prove to be more than enough for someone else.

Chapter 21

There Are Days When Time Stands Still

How to be honest with yourself and open to those around you.

The hands of the clock don't seem to move as fast and everything spins in slow motion. Seconds could feel like a month. Minutes might feel like a year. Whatever the situation is, however, we may or may not want those days to last.

We might not want to feel the heartache that brought us those long days, but we know it's there. We eventually have to confront it – not just deal with it so it goes away for a while. There might even be a moment when we have to not only be honest with ourselves, but also be open to others around us.

It's a moment when we must not only feel pain, but also acknowledge it. That's when we find out exactly where we place honesty on our scale of importance. It might not land on the spot we wanted or expected. Or it may land perfectly. Either way, we re-learn things we thought we knew all along.

I thought the notion of death wouldn't hit me as hard as it did with my grandfather. I thought going through the process of losing someone whom I was close to would be what I'd always been told it was: saying goodbye to that person while they're sleeping. I didn't know any better, so I didn't question it. I'd only been to a handful of funerals up until his passing, but something was different this time.

I was old enough to understand what was actually going on. My grandfather was not sleeping, nor was he coming back. There was nothing anyone could do or say that would change that, no magic wand to wave. All I knew at this moment was that I needed something – a wave, a faint smile, a nod – to let me know things were going to be OK. They were far from that at the time, and I knew it would take a long time before life would feel normal again. Or whatever my family would come to know as normal.

I wasn't sure that day would ever come. I also tried to make sense of the fact that this great man was the first of my grandparents to be laid to rest. Why did this happen? Did someone else need him more than my family?

I wrestled with this in the few short days leading up to his funeral as I thought about all of the plans I had for my future, and the ambitions that I had of becoming "the best writer in the world," as my grandparents always told everyone they crossed paths with. So, here I was – one year away from graduating high school and having my priorities rearranged in a shocking, painful way. Everything came to a screeching, sudden halt – and I stopped with it. So did my entire family, including my younger brother who my parents had adopted three years before this tragedy struck.

He was too young to realize what had happened and why we were preparing to say goodbye to someone he barely got to know. It wasn't fair that his time with him was so short, but this entire situation wasn't fair to any of us. My older brother, however, knew what was going on like I did. I could tell he was numb from the sadness and shock, but he was trying his best to be strong for everyone.

I didn't want anyone to know that this was all crashing down around me, but I couldn't hide my own sadness. I was trying to catch these now shattered pieces of my life as they fell. When the day came to say goodbye, my family did everything they could to not fall apart. My parents quietly loaded me into our van and made sure everyone was as comfortable as possible.

We arrived at the funeral home later that day to find many of our family members who live out of town quietly gathered in a well-lit hallway – hugging and crying on each other's shoulders. I waited there with my parents because I was too devastated to go into the next room where the casket was. My older brother went in to comfort my nana, who was already there. My uncle and aunt met us in the hallway and cried with us.

I was close enough to the door to peak in, and saw that the casket was open. My heart immediately sunk and my hands started to sweat. As I tried to gather myself, a long line of my grandfather's friends, acquaintances and longtime co-workers began to form. It wrapped around the outside of the funeral home and seemingly went on for miles. It was fitting, because my grandfather knew almost everyone in town.

The line kept getting longer as my mom, uncle and aunt – his and my nana's children – walked into the room to greet and thank the hundreds of people who came to pay their respects. Every person who passed by the casket stopped to share a deep embrace with Nana, who had been crying for so long that her tears dried on her face. I slowly went into the room, in amongst the quiet chaos, -- when I saw someone hug my mom before politely making her way through the crowd to get to me.

She came closer and smiled. I broke down right away, because this wasn't a stranger. This was my one of my best friends, Rachel, who was in many of my classes and could make me laugh on my worst day. She didn't say anything as she was now standing in front of me. She just hugged me until I calmed down.

I knew two things right then and there: I was going to be OK and most importantly, I had a genuine best friend.

Both things are still true, more than 15 years later.

Life isn't always fair, but there is always a reason to be honest with yourself. It may not come easily and take more work than you're prepared for. When you have loving, caring people in your corner, however, you can't go wrong!

Chapter 22

Where Are the Loyal?

We find out who our true friends are when our backs are against the wall.

We may have compassionate people around us when we're at our lowest, but not fully embrace the fact they're in our corner. Or it can be the complete opposite.

We could be in the fight of our lives and have no one there to support us. Some people might see us struggling – or even know what we're going through – and not bother to lend a helping hand. What we have to realize, however, it's their choice to not be there. We might not agree with it, but it's still their decision. And theirs alone.

It's at this very moment when we have to stop, take a look around and ask ourselves, *Who's really been here all along?* and *What truly matters?*

That's exactly what I did in the months leading up to my senior year of high school. I'd been fighting a mostly quiet fight of self-discovery and acceptance by myself for so long. I taught myself how to fight for everything I had.

I was so accustomed to fighting on my own I wasn't sure how to react when people started coming into my life naturally, instead of having to step in to help me with something. My cerebral palsy dictated my life in that manner, and I didn't want to scare anyone away. Not only that, but I was still riding a wave of raw emotion from the events that suddenly unfolded in my life.

I tried to remember the good times, the sun-filled days with ice cream and smiles. I remembered the valuable way I was taught to look at my disability, and how my family always reinforced it. Now, I had people with new, refreshing attitudes around me. They were my peers at school, who weren't interested in hearing every excruciating detail of life as I knew it, and didn't mind not knowing about that part of my journey. That admittedly took me by surprise, mainly because it reminded me of how I was raised.

The fact that my classmates were treating me with that kind of respect was great. It felt like a weight had been lifted off my shoulders, but I was fully aware that it didn't happen overnight.

The rest of my peers, however, didn't take exception to my disability at all. They read my name in the school newspaper every few weeks and had gotten used to reading my articles as well. I hoped, as I always did when my words were read by anyone, it would be a reason for my classmates to think of me as one of their peers. Just like I thought of them as mine.

As luck would have it, that's exactly what happened. Everyone slowly came to know me as "the writer" in school – giving me an occasional high five and telling me I was cool. I never dreamed of being the coolest kid at my high school. Nor did I want to be, but I took in stride because I now felt confident my classmates knew I was one of them.

I also felt like I was in the same boat they were in – getting through their last few years of mandatory schooling before moving on to whatever was next. The best part was they wanted to get to know me. I didn't take it as them wanting to be best friends for life, however. I instead looked at it as a gesture of kindness and genuine curiosity on their part. For me, it was a way of healing and getting my life back on track after my grandfather's death.

I'd made a few friends in tenth and eleventh grade – whom I'm still friends with today – that didn't ask about what happened. They didn't try to dig into my past, either. It got to the point where they would say, "Stop!" when I started talking about it. I slowly learned it wasn't because they didn't care. They simply didn't take any interest in basing our friendship on my cerebral palsy.

I knew I didn't have to worry about Rachel, because she had been there for me since the very first few days of high school – and proved she was a loyal friend more times than I can count. Even so, I still struggled to be OK with people coming into my life. Waves of uncertainty began rolling in, and I tried to ignore them. It all brought me back to my classroom in sixth grade, where I got my heart broken when someone who I thought was my sidekick stabbed me in the back.

"Erin, I can't be friends with you anymore," he said.

Confused, I took a minute to figure out why a friend of at least six years would suddenly be telling me this. I couldn't come up with a good reason, so I said the only logical thing I could say: "Why?"

"Well, we're going into junior high next year. I can't be seen hanging around someone in a wheelchair."

I was stunned. I sat there for a while and thought about the words that had just come out of his mouth. I didn't lie to myself. I didn't try to change his mind, either. I decided this so-called "friend" wasn't worth my tears, even though I was devastated. I said goodbye and never looked back.

It took me years to be comfortable with myself again. In fact, I didn't tell my parents about this until a year after the fact. I was too wounded, but this experience helped me realize why I shouldn't be ashamed to tell others how I feel.

Sometimes that's all it takes. Sometimes you have to be broken before you find out what you're truly worth.

When you put yourself back together, however, you'll find you are enough. And always will be.

Chapter 23

What Is a Worthwhile Moment?

The benefits might not be all about you.

The human race is an interesting blend of hope, excitement, uncertainty, and ambition. We all have somewhere we want to be in life. We all have a destination that may be miles away from where we are or just a few steps away.

It seems like we're always searching for something more, regardless of how successful or comfortable we become. It may be rewarding when we arrive at that place we think we've found everything we're looking for. It might even feel surreal or sublime for a certain period of time, but still, a part of us isn't satisfied.

The search then becomes one of personal needs, wants and perhaps even selfishness. We get what we want, but at what cost? We have to decide if it's worth staying in a comfortable spot or move on to something new. Or stay where we are and try to make do with what we have.

My senior year of high school posed these questions more than once and in many ways. It felt as if a different part of my soul was being put under a microscope every time. These weren't the questions I'd tried to find answers to up until this point. They were new ones that suddenly had a heartbeat – and they couldn't simply be swept under the rug.

Things had been so scary and uncertain that I almost forgot to breathe. I was getting to a comfortable place in my life but wasn't quite there yet. I needed to learn how to turn rejection and pain into something I could use to better myself. I'd had enough of both to know what it felt like when they stay with you longer than a little while.

I didn't know what to do with those emotions.

I had to balance this while parting ways with certain people in my life – including my personal care aides I had throughout junior high and high school, who helped me in class as well as getting me through what I considered a typical school day. This included everything from taking notes in each class to helping me with my lunch. They were truly instrumental in making sure I got the most out of my education without having to put too much focus on my cerebral palsy. Even though I had all of this swirling around me, I was still searching for some stability.

I had answers, but they weren't what I was hoping for.

My dream of being a writer would have to remain a long-term goal, and I made peace with that. I wished my friends well and hoped the bonds we made would last. Little did I know, graduation day itself would provide a sense of stability I never had before.

All my classmates were getting ready when the big day finally arrived. I was getting ready, too, but in my own way. We gathered in the outdoor athletic complex where many events were held. As family members and guests began to fill every seat, my hands started to sweat and my mind was racing.

No one knew I was about to get out of my wheelchair and walk across a makeshift stage to receive my diploma. I had been secretly practicing and planning for months with my walker, but kept it within a small circle of people who helped me see this through, including my family. It was my idea, and I wanted it to be special.

The ceremony started with greetings and warm wishes before the emcee introduced my graduating class. I patiently waited for each name to be announced, knowing what was going to happen. In truth, I was grateful my name didn't start with an A. I still had a few minutes to gather myself and try to calm my nerves, which didn't work out so well. My personal care aide helped me get in position in my walker as last names starting with I and J were called.

I was as ready as I was going to be by the time the emcee got to the letter K. My name was announced a few minutes later as complete silence fell over the crowd. Everyone gasped and wondered why there was such a long pause. Then, they caught a glimpse of me and slowly realized what was going on. I looked up to see my family crying a flood of joyful tears, especially my dad.

The crowd erupted into a standing ovation when I emerged in my walker. I was completely exhausted between calming myself and trudging through a long strip of thick grass. I made my way on stage, accepted my diploma.

The celebration continued for what seemed like 10 to 15 minutes before moving on with the ceremony. I couldn't help but think I didn't deserve this. All I did was what I'd been telling myself I was going to do for months. I wondered if it would have any impact on anyone. As I stood there looking out into the massive sea of humanity, I didn't have to wonder anymore.

I did what I set out to do and more.

I realized my actions did something fulfilling – not only for myself but for everyone who was there that day. My hope is that they were able to take something worthwhile with them, the same way I have.

When you're going through life, decide if it's truly all about yourself. Or if it's about showing others something from a new perspective. Decide what kind of person you want to be, and go be it the best way you know how.

Chapter 24

Realize the Potential

Some things are too big to be put in a box.

Potential can be a wonderful, prosperous thing. It can take to heights others may consider unattainable or unrealistic. We might even be able to help someone who doesn't see potential – in themselves or anything around them.

We might even see it in ourselves unless someone else takes the time to pull it out of us. Sometimes we recognize we have something special inside, but don't know what to do with it. Or even know how to present it to others in a subtle, confident way.

This was one of my biggest hurdles in the weeks and months following high school, on the heels of sharing a very unexpected but worthwhile moment with my family and a crowd full of other proud family members who came to graduation. I graduated with a quiet confidence in myself, as well as the ability to write. I started thinking logically about how I might be able to utilize it in whatever I'd decide to do on a long or short-term basis.

It was a level of confidence I hadn't felt in a long time. So much so I had to re-acquaint myself with it. I was almost afraid of it because it felt like I was headed in the direction I always wanted to be in. Not only that, but it felt strange – almost dangerous – to associate that feeling with anything other than my cerebral palsy.

I had spent so much time getting used to my disability over the years, it was difficult to completely remove it from any given situation. It made me feel unstable in many ways – and again, I didn't know what to do with my sense of insecurity.

That's not to say I didn't want my disability to be an entirely separate entity. I always wanted that more than anyone knew. I realized as I got older, however, my cerebral palsy, and everything that came with it, was always going to be intertwined with every aspect of my existence. It was even more obvious at this particular point in time, as I was fresh out of high school and looking ahead to what was next.

Graduating gave me an opportunity to think about certain things individually. It also allowed me to truly consider how I wanted to carve out a path for myself, and how it would impact others. If anything, writing would become a bridge over one of the biggest gaps in my life. I couldn't separate my disability from everything else in my world, so I decided I wanted to blend the two together. I didn't know how or when it would happen. I knew if there was a way to do it, I was going to find it.

Like many times before, however, I didn't have any ties to published authors or anyone influential in the writing industry. That bothered me when I was simply daydreaming about a career, but it quickly became apparent it was the one thing that had been missing all this time. I was confident it was the difference between simply expressing myself and conveying an important message to an audience other than my family and friends.

I needed – and really wanted – someone to show me how to balance, hoping to build upon the many years I spent writing. With high school in the rearview mirror, I did the one thing I thought would help me meet most of my short-term goals: apply to college. This had not only a personal goal itself, but it was now something I felt I had to do. I wasn't even close to being the polished writer I wanted to be, so the thought of going to college became my motivation to keep moving forward.

It was a welcomed beam of light because I did what I needed to do – and put in the time – to arrive at the threshold of this decision. I planned on making the most of every lesson I learned. I also hoped the fact I did work hard to graduate would shine through when I applied to different colleges.

I ended up applying to a few, including Penn State Altoona, a full-service branch campus of Pennsylvania State University. It was very close to home, which I appreciated in my own unique way. There were two very big factors that really drew me in, however: this campus had the accessibility I needed and the classes I wanted.

The spring before high school graduation was filled with anticipation as my family and I waited to find out if I had been accepted at any of the colleges I applied to. It was a much longer process than we anticipated due to my disability, but it provided the stability I was looking for as I was accepted at Penn State Altoona in Fall 2004.

My first thoughts upon receiving this amazing news were, *This is real now!* and *Have I made my family proud?* I wasn't worried about fitting in or being accepted by my professors and peers. I knew that would be a work in progress. I didn't realize how smooth and relatively quick the transition would be, however. Nor did I fully consider the fact that I wasn't going to be in classrooms with little kids anymore. I was going to be around mature, open-minded people. At least, I hoped that would be the case.

All I had when I arrived at Penn State Altoona was my passion for writing. I simply put it on the table and made sure my cerebral palsy wasn't in the way, I wanted everyone there to see my abilities – and they did. Little did I know, my life was about to change in the best ways possible.

Some things are too big to be put in a box. You may be able to keep them there for a while and maybe fit more things in. Then it gets too full. You don't realize how much you've piled on top of the important things until you sort things out. You might even find something that wasn't meant to be put in a box in the first place.

Chapter 25

Take a Chance on Yourself

Are you ready to show the world what you can do?

Abraham Lincoln said, "Actions speak louder than words." I have found that our actions may not have an impact right away. They might not even mean anything to anyone until they have a genuine purpose behind them.

Some say it's all about timing things right. Others say it's about having the right people behind us and our cause. Then, there are those who believe we need to be in the right place at the right time before something worthwhile happens. These ways of thinking hold a certain power and truth on their own – and they're wise words to live by.

As I'd find out, however, something absolutely magical happens when all three are combined with one mindset— our actions will define who we are.

I wasn't sure what to expect going into my freshman year of college. I didn't expect to get a letter in the mail notifying me I had been accepted at Penn State Altoona. It happened rather quickly. I didn't feel like anything I'd done in my life particularly defined me, either – at least not in terms of making career choices or turning my passion for writing into something viable with a genuine heartbeat other people could feel.

That happened with time. It would be an uphill battle, even if I didn't have a disability. The fact I've never been without extra pressure motivated me. It helped me figure out how I wanted to approach my professors, as well as what kind of impression I wanted to put out there. It was very important to me that I showed them something other than the obvious – something they might not have known or guessed by looking at me.

If anything, I wanted to see if the choices and decisions I'd made up to this point were truly the right ones. Or close to being what I thought was right. I wasn't terribly worried about anything else. I knew questions and concerns about my cerebral palsy would arise naturally, and I told myself they would be handled in the same manner. I wanted to believe Penn State Altoona was a place in which any judgments could be left at the door. I wanted it to be the place where I somehow bridged the gap between my writing and my disability. I was excited about the opportunity to start a new chapter in my life. I didn't think it would open with a question like, "Have you considered writing as a career?"

I was only a few months into my freshman year. One of my English professors calmly pulled me aside after class one day and asked me this – perhaps the most crucial question I've ever been asked. There was no pause. No hesitation. There was a level of direct certainty and intention I had never heard before.

I swallowed hard. "Yes, that has been my dream ever since I was a little kid."

A big smile crept across my professor's face. I wasn't sure exactly what it meant, but I knew enough to know it was genuine. I also had a strong feeling that this smile was coming from someone who already arrived at the place I wanted to be career-wise – and had been there enough times to know what they were doing.

It didn't even cross my mind I'd been turning in well-written assignments. I gave my best no matter what I wrote or whom it was for. In this particular moment, my best was enough to give someone who would become very influential in my life, a reason to pause. It was the first time I didn't have to explain myself or feel like I was being put underneath a microscope because of things I couldn't control.

It felt great and I was determined to build upon this beautiful moment. I immediately wanted to make sure this professor – and every professor I'd have for all of my classes – knew I took writing seriously. I also had my mind set on making sure they weren't wasting their time on me. That meant pouring my heart on paper, and most importantly, working harder than I'd ever worked before.

This was the start of something wonderful. I felt in my bones and deep down in my soul. If no one else knew it, I was going to show them. This was all on me – and I gave it all I had because it truly mattered now.

Sometimes an opportunity presents itself for you to shine. It may feel heavier than your shoulders can take. It may even feel a little awkward and unexpected, but that's the moment when you kick the door down and show the world what you can truly do, when you give yourself a chance.

Chapter 26

There's a Time and a Place for Everything

Though, it might not look or feel like it sometimes.

Our situation may not be ideal. It might be a matter of putting all our chips on the table and seeing what unfolds. Or there could be something hidden beneath the surface starting to shine.

It might take a while for others to see its worth, but time could also be the thing to motivate us. We continue traveling down our paths – whatever they might be – not realizing we're doing something worthy of being respected or admired. Then, people begin to pay attention for the right reasons. Heads slowly start to turn and there's a sense of responsibility on our part, to not only live up to our own standards but those of people who have put any amount of faith in us as well

There are no words when the moment arrives. There's only a tremendous amount of gratitude, which I felt as I started to ease into life as a college student. I continued turning in what I thought were clean, well-written assignments. I didn't think they were masterpieces or works of art, but I didn't think they were sloppy, either.

I wanted to see what would happen if I stayed on this path, given the fact that one of my professors noticed something important without me having to draw attention to it. The moment lit a fire underneath me because it was pure and genuine. More importantly, it wasn't based on my disability.

I wanted to have more moments like that. In the back of my mind, there wasn't a better place than Penn State Altoona to create such meaningful moments. I looked at every assignment as a reason to show my professors I belonged where I was. I also tried to soak in every bit of feedback or wise words they sent my way.

I wanted to learn everything I could about writing because it was a world I had been exploring for as long as I could remember. I told myself, 'Just keep doing what you're doing and you'll be fine. They'll see what you're trying to show them in due time. Part of this was because I had something to prove like I always have. Along the way, however, I started to get a deeper sense that something monumental was happening.

My professors didn't cater to me. They didn't make the assignments easier or talk to me like I had no idea what I was doing in their classes. I tried to keep in mind that they didn't know what to expect when I rolled in. They had every right to believe I wasn't worth their time, and I wouldn't have been shocked or offended if they did.

They fortunately didn't, as they treated me the way I had always wanted to be treated – especially by people I didn't know or didn't know me. If anything, it was the way I'd always been told I should be treated. They showed a level of compassion and professionalism that truly allowed me to find out who and what I was meant to be.

They didn't question my abilities. They simply let me spread my wings. I'm sure there was some uncertainty below the surface, but I never saw it. It felt as if they held the key to loosen the chains I carried for so long. I didn't want to let it slip through my fingers – and they would make sure I earned it.

I knew my professors weren't complimenting me simply for the sake of saying nice, positive things. They were paying much closer attention than I thought they were – and it wasn't because they felt pity for me. In fact, it was the complete opposite.

I was sitting in one of my English classes, working on an outline for an assigned essay, when I heard, "Erin, you've got magic in your fingers!" I looked up to see another one of my professors quietly reading what I'd written so far.

That alone made me feel like everything I did before college wasn't a waste. I never felt like I had to earn the right to be treated like a normal human being, but this was suddenly a clear validation of why I should have felt that way all along. In this moment, however. it was more than a simple feeling of *I'm really grateful to be here!*

It was even more than knowing I had a real opportunity to do something worthwhile with my life. The feeling was rushing through my body was one of personal truth – a certainty arose. This part of my journey was not going to be a free ride because of my shortcomings and preconceived disadvantages.

I didn't expect to be. I'd never gotten a pass because of my cerebral palsy before. I wasn't about to give anyone a reason to think I needed one now. I came too far and worked too hard to show people the wrong things at this point.

It wasn't a matter of now or never. It was a way for me to continue earning what my professors gave me – whether it was advice, praise, or respect.

If you do something for the sake of doing it, you might get some attention. If you do it with purpose, however, people are bound to take notice. Whatever you do, however, do it because it matters.

Chapter 27

Center the Inner Force

It could be the best thing or the worst for ourselves.

The universe has a unique way of telling us what we need, and when we need it. Sometimes it's like a gentle nudge from something someone says or does. Other times, finding out what we need is not about external nudges at all.

Our needs can be nudged by how we feel inside. Or how we choose to think, so we can move forward. Whatever the inner force is, it's always very real and present. It's up to us to do everything we can to use it in a positive way, which can turn out to be the best or worst thing we do for ourselves.

I've always been determined to utilize what I have in a positive manner. Or at least in a way to help me understand why it's me who's in a wheelchair instead of someone else. I was in the middle of my freshman year at Penn State Altoona when I discovered something that would fuel my desire to pursue a career as a writer even more. It was subtle and quiet at first but spun into a wild whirlwind of emotion I could barely control or ignore by the end of the year.

My professors continued to notice my passion for writing. I was thrilled — not only because I wasn't being looked at as "the girl in a wheelchair", but also because all of this was happening naturally. It didn't feel forced, so I made a personal commitment to work twice as hard as anyone expected of me.

I made it my mission to keep pouring my heart into everything that came across my professors' desks to show them I was paying as much attention as they were. I put a lot of pressure on myself, but I always have done that regardless of whatever situation or setting I'm in. It was more about keeping my momentum going. Not only that, but I knew I had the attention of the right people. The fact that I earned it in my own way was even more motivation to do my absolute best.

As all of this was unfolding, however, I realized my chains had been loosened enough and I could let my soul breathe. The chains weren't gone, I just didn't let them control me. I started to feel differently about my circumstances. I wanted to get away from centering everything around my disability. Or as far away as my cerebral palsy would allow.

I knew it wouldn't be realistic to completely disregard or deny the fact I've been dealt a very specific hand of cards. I also knew my life would not have had a chance without that set of cards. At least not up until this point. Most importantly, however, I had finally come to terms with the notion that these were the cold, hard facts of my existence. There was less room for doubt now.

There was no way I could have changed any of this, even if I wanted to. I simply wanted there to be some space between my immediate reality and the world my writing was creating. My new surroundings in college were the opening I'd always hoped for, so I set my mind on making sure it stayed wide open.

My younger self would not have known what to do at this moment. Maybe she would've felt like her circumstances were too much to handle, and she was still trying to find her place in the world. She would've said, *I'll find a way!*, even if she didn't know where she was going or what to make of the opportunities that were in front of her.

My older self said the same thing. The only difference was I had a destination in sight – and there weren't any unexpected obstacles in the way. There was only a genuine sense of getting somewhere. Another step toward creating the very personal space I now wanted.

We all start out in certain places with certain goals and ideas. Then, things happen to help you realize that you have other aspirations, too. It doesn't mean you have to throw away the ones you started. It means your story is uniquely yours to tell, and sometimes there's more to it than meets the eye.

Chapter 28

Lift Another and Elevate Yourself

The world often seems small.

It can make us feel like we're in our own little bubble and no one is paying any attention. It might even feel like we're carrying the weight of the world itself on our shoulders.

We do our best to make ends meet, but it never seems to be enough. Either something doesn't measure up to someone else's standards, or someone else cuts to the front of the line so they can reap another person's benefits. That's the moment when we have to ask ourselves, *What kind of human being do I want others to see in me?* and *What do I want people to remember?*

I was thinking about the answers to both of these questions as I made my way through college. I felt confident I was being treated equally and people on campus weren't looking at my wheelchair. They were looking past it, which felt better than I ever imagined it would.

A significant amount of weight had been lifted off my shoulders without me having to say, *I have cerebral palsy.* I wanted to try to shed that weight completely. If I couldn't, I wanted to continue to use my passion for writing as a motivation to show others what I was capable of. Not only that, but I was starting to earn the respect of my peers in college as well.

I began wondering, *If my writing can make that kind of impact here, what else could it do in an even bigger setting? How many more people would be willing to read what I write, and how would they take it?* I wasn't interested in making people feel bad for me. I couldn't hide my disability any better now than when I was younger, so there was no point in trying. I wasn't looking to radically change anyone's minds about me or my circumstances, either.

The biggest thing I wanted at this point was for everyone to see the real me. I didn't give much thought to anything else. I knew convincing "everyone" to see past my disability would be a gigantic feat, but I still felt like I had a responsibility to give others something to think about. I thought more people could make up their own minds if I gave them enough of myself.

If I continued to put myself out there through my writing, I knew everything else would come naturally – just like it had been in the few short months since arriving at Penn State Altoona. It wasn't until I started crossing paths with people who had drastically different stories than mine, I realized how small my problems and worries truly were. They were people who have scratched, clawed, fought and struggled their entire lives. Many of them are still fighting, but have yet to give up.

There was a sharp, immediate sense they were cut from the same cloth as I was, as I learned more about them and their stories. I had no right to complain about anything in my life after hearing why these people were the way they were – from fighting cancer battles to choosing to travel halfway around the world to attend college and inadvertently build a new life and everything in between. I had no right to judge these people, either – and I didn't. I knew the feeling of being judged all too well and wasn't going to cast that shadow on them.

If anything, I hoped to be some small source of light for them. I had never known or heard of anyone who could not only crawl out of such deep, dark holes but also had the strength and resolve to rise from their circumstances so brilliantly and courageously. I felt like my writing was something I could offer them, to let them know they weren't alone. And to also let them know they had a confidante in me if they ever chose to reach out.

I admittedly felt selfish for deeming my personal problems as heavy and troublesome. I asked myself at that moment, *What kind of person would I be if I gave up an opportunity to be something for someone else? Would I still have a chance to inspire others if I didn't have cerebral palsy?*

I thought about it a lot. And still do. I also thought about whether or not the people I met in college would still want to be a part of my life after we graduated and moved on. Through thick, thin and some of the best years of my life, I don't have to wonder anymore.

Never turn down an opportunity to lift someone up. You might be surprised what you learn about them – and yourself.

Chapter 29

Burdens To Bear

We all want good things in life.

We all hope that prosperity, whether it's financial, personal or the latter, will come out of those things if we do them right and work hard.

We might follow in someone's footsteps. Or go off the beaten path, where something better could be waiting for us. When we do that, however, it's more than a calculated risk or a snap decision. It's a statement to let those around us know we want more than what we've found or have been provided.

It's not always a measure of spite or revenge for things that may have gone wrong. Nor is it a constant bundle of negative feelings. It can be a release – a realization we don't have the right to judge or place our burdens onto other people, especially those whom we treasure the most.

College helped me see there's more to being gentle, kind and strong than meets the eye. I kept crossing paths with people who were nothing like me on the surface. Yet, there was still an instant, almost automatic feeling I had more in common with them than I did with anyone else I had met so far. We ended up taking many of the same classes together, so I was at ease asking for help when I needed it.

They took notes for me, held doors open and even walked me to my mom's car after class every day. At the same time, however, they never assumed I always wanted or needed help. They knew there were certain things they had to do for me – like getting my books out of my bookbag – but they also quickly picked up on the things I could do on my own. I was extremely grateful they recognized the fact I needed personal space.

It was never a matter of, "If you scratch my back, I'll scratch yours!' It was always based on trust – and most importantly, mutual respect. I felt strangely comfortable around my new friends, and they felt comfortable around me as we continued to have classes together every semester. I knew they all had heavy burdens to bear.

I didn't want to dig into that unless they were willing to share. In turn, I didn't have to explain why I'm in a wheelchair. They rarely asked. When they did, however, it wasn't because they saw something "wrong" with me. They asked out of genuine compassion and curiosity, which I appreciated even more. As our friendships grew, however, I didn't want them to feel like they had to take care of me.

I didn't want them to worry about helping me carry the burden of having a disability. My disability has always been my load to carry, and it wasn't fair to put it on their shoulders. Or ask them to take on the responsibility. Nor did I want to make them feel like I was trying to get something from them by having them in my life. I don't think they ever felt that way, but I still had a sense I had to avoid it at all costs.

I thought about that a lot because it was unfamiliar territory for me. I had waited too long to have these types of friends. I didn't know if I would again, so I was going to keep them close – if they wanted me in their lives. I was so used to explaining the same part of my story to everyone I met, I didn't know what it felt like to leave my disability out of any conversation. It got to the point where my newfound buddies would tell me, "I don't want to hear about that." – not because they didn't care, but because they didn't see my disability as a reason to stay by my side.

They had my back because they wanted to. They saw the full portrait of the fighter and writer the rest of the world was beginning to see. It was liberating to know I didn't have to be defensive about my disability anymore – at least, not around these friends.

It wasn't until one of them looked me in the eye and said, "You know, I'd switch places with you any time, Erin!" then I realized how incredibly fortunate I was to even know these people who were random strangers six months to a year before crossing paths in the first place.

It might take people a long time to see the beauty in something. They might not turn the corner at the same time everyone else does – but when they do, make it worth their time.

Chapter 30

Momentum Motivates

Keep yourself moving toward the goal when nothing else will push you.

The word "best" is often associated with many things in life. Best house. Best car. Best friend. The list is seemingly endless. We all have our opinions about what the best things in the world are. Or what we think the next best thing will be.

Whatever we attach to that word, however, has a tendency to become an expectation. We expect that person, place or thing to always be a certain way – and make us think or feel a certain way in the process. We often stumble upon something that tests our claims about what we think the ultimate "best" truly is. When we're proven wrong, we can either deny it or find a way to make the situation better.

I've always looked at myself as a normal person. I don't think my cerebral palsy makes me "special", and I refuse to carry myself in such a manner. While I put my heart and soul into everything I do, I'd like to think I'm no different than anyone else who's trying to live a decent life. I'm also aware that dealing with cerebral palsy is a part of my everyday life. I don't see it as something out of the ordinary or an obstacle I have to overcome because it's always going to stay with me. It is, however, a vital, substantial part of my existence – just like writing is.

I might be a good writer, but being good doesn't give me the right to gloat or force people to read a single word I write. Nor do I have the right to make others feel the same way I do. Or make them think my circumstances alone make me worthy of any kind of praise.

I began to pay a lot more attention to how I carried myself as I entered adulthood. I also thought about the message I was sending through my actions, and what impact it had on others.

I was on the cusp of starting the second half of my Bachelor's degree in college, but other things outside of my academics were bubbling to the surface.

I started to sense that what I was doing resonated with people. Some stopped to take a second glance. Others told me, "I hope you know you inspire me!" I'd be driving my wheelchair down the hall on my way to class when this would happen – or strategically maneuvering my chair so I could fit through a door halfway open. People were kind enough to stop and help, but it felt strange – yet quite flattering – being called an inspiration for doing things that weren't outside the range of my capabilities.

I didn't know how to react or respond at first. I was simply trying to get through college and make the most of it along the way. It wasn't my initial goal to motivate or inspire anyone, but I slowly realized it was a built-in responsibility. As long as I remained consciously aware, I was going to use it for something good and positive.

In the midst of all this, I joined the staff of Penn State Altoona's newspaper – which proved to be another big step in the right direction. Everyone – my peers, classmates, and professors were still stopping me in hallways on campus. Now, however, were calling my writing inspirational. I was shocked and humbled at the same time. It never occurred to me I might have done something someone else deemed inspirational.

Someone stopped me again and said, "You're the best writer this newspaper has had in years!" I now knew I had done something truly powerful, and the things that made me unique had nothing to do with my physical circumstances.

I was so used to doing everything with the extra weight of my disability attached to it. This wasn't anything new, but I guess people looked at my life from a different angle – and still do. Maybe they say to themselves, 'If she can live life and still overcome her obstacles, so can I.'

I had the respect I had always hoped to earn, along with the strong but gentle friends I thought I'd never have. Now, however, it was more about keeping this momentum going than anything else.

When you have momentum on your side, do everything you can to keep it. It will be what motivates you when nothing else does. Most importantly, it will help you get to the top of whatever mountain you're climbing.

Chapter 31

Dig Deep and Drown the Noise the World Makes

When confidence is crushed by a lack of control.

It's hard to predict what's next in life. We often think we have a tight grip on the next hour, day, month or even year. Then reality hits. We start to see how much control we've lost constantly trying to be in control of our time, money and seemingly everything else we have the power to manipulate.

It's a continuous cycle which society functions upon – and gives us signals that it's acceptable or healthy to think we can control everything around us. What if, however, we gave up a little bit of madness? What if we simply allowed things to happen, instead of always trying to force a situation to unfold or be resolved the way we want?

It was abundantly clear things were working in my favor when my sophomore year of college began. I had everything I wanted. Most importantly, I earned everything that came my way. I was riding a wave of momentum, but I had a feeling the rest of my college career couldn't go as smoothly as it had been. Something had gone wrong or gotten in my way because that's how I've always dealt with life.

I wasn't hoping for anything to go wrong. Nor was I trying to let negative thoughts creep into my head. It all felt too good to be true, but I continued to enjoy the things I had worked for. I knew other people noticed I wasn't "showing off" or simply aiming to get good grades. I was working hard because it was all I knew how to do – and I was now surrounded by published authors and writers who had already been to the top of the mountain I was climbing.

I've always known my disability doesn't allow me to control many aspects of my own life. This, however, was something I did have full control over. I wasn't going to let the wealth of knowledge from my professors slip through my fingers.

Not only that, but I wanted to prove to myself I could become the writer I always wanted to be. I slowly realized I was inadvertently crossing big things off of a list I never intended to write. These were things – like making worthwhile friendships and legitimately thinking about a life outside the realm of my cerebral palsy – that I would have shrugged off when I was younger. They felt so far away back then they almost didn't seem real.

Yet, here I was – getting closer to finishing my sophomore year at Penn State Altoona. I had two more years to go and began asking myself, 'What's going to happen after I graduate?' and 'Who's going to hire me?' I couldn't stop thinking about those two things, because it was an uphill battle getting to the point where I could even consider attending college. I wanted everything I'd do after this – and every person I'd meet – to have a special place in my life.

It was around this time when I met with a caseworker from an organization in my hometown of Altoona, PA. The organization aimed to help people with disabilities find steady employment. The caseworker whom I met with, however, was not convinced a career as a writer was the right thing to pursue. I was told it wasn't a profitable decision, and I would never "make it" in the writing industry.

I was used to doubt. I was used to being told "no", but this was my first time being completely shunned by someone who was supposed to help me. Moreover, I had never been told I couldn't "be" something prior to this moment. Part of me expected this kind of treatment. Another part wanted to scream.

My confidence was crushed, but I kept going. I thought I was in the process of crossing another thing off my list by continuing with college when I was called into the Admissions Office at Penn State Altoona with my parents.

"Erin, we need to have a meeting right away," the woman in charge of disability services on campus said.

"OK," I replied, dumbfounded and confused. "What's the meeting about?"

I maneuvered my wheelchair into a conference room to find my caseworker sitting there – with papers in front of her. I flipped the power button to my motor off and got as comfortable as I could.

My parents had sat down, as my caseworker proceeded to inform us it was time for me to get a job.

And I needed to leave college right then and there.

There was a mass of dead, thick air in the room as these words came out of her mouth. I didn't say anything, because I didn't know what to say. My parents, on the other hand, reacted with swift emotion.

"I don't understand," my mom chimed in, trying not to let her anger show. "Why do you want Erin to do this?"

"Well, she's been in college for two years and hasn't found employment yet."

My parents fought this tooth and nail. I was distraught, but I listened. I left Penn State Altoona at the end of my sophomore year, graduating with an Associate's degree in 2006. My hope was to get hired at a suitable job. The biggest problem was all the positions I applied for focused on quantity of work instead of quality. I had the efficiency, but not the speed.

I was at my wit's end a year later. I was getting rejected at every turn, leaving me mentally exhausted. Little did I know, my next major decision would change my life again – even more than I thought possible.

You may not have all the control you want. You might not even know what to do with the control you have. At some point, you have to dig deep and drown out the noise the world makes. Your heart is the only thing you truly must listen to.

Chapter 32

Don't Let Them Tear You Down

There will always be naysayers in the crowd.

The universe has its own unique way of telling us when something isn't meant to be. It may come in the form of a harsh word, misinterpretation or a blatant lie. We sometimes tell ourselves that it's a simple misunderstanding – and the person who stooped to an unbelievable low didn't intend to go that far.

We might even want to forgive them. Or let their words and actions sink in before pointing fingers and making false judgments. What if we're perceptive enough to know the person on the other end is making us feel so small it's like we don't exist? Most importantly, what if we respect ourselves enough to believe the truth when it's disguised as a beautiful lie?

I didn't want to tell myself the truth when I was struggling to find a job in 2007. I didn't want to believe I was forced to drop out of college. Nor could I bear the fact I finally listened to someone else's plan for my life and was cheated out of my education in return. All the while, I kept knocking on employers' doors. And kept getting rejected.

"We're sorry, you're not what we're looking for."

"We want employees who have speed. You're not fast enough."

My back was against the wall. It wasn't like I'd never been knocked down before, but I felt trapped this time. I knew my hands were tied during that meeting with my caseworker and my parents at Penn State Altoona in 2006, before starting my reluctant job search. Not only that, but I now knew there was someone in the world who didn't want me to succeed in life. At least not as a writer.

There was nothing the staff or my parents could do during that meeting, either – which made me feel even more worthless. In fact, the baffled, almost defensive look on the face of every staff member in attendance told the entire story. I was on the Honor Roll for most of my sophomore year, and even for part of my freshman year. No one in that room could understand why I was being forced to give up everything I had worked for until this point when my grades spoke for themselves.

The fact this all came about because of someone who was hired to help me continue on my chosen path made my stomach turn. I wasn't asking for a hand-out. I didn't even know there was a problem until my parents and I were abruptly called into the conference room in the first place.

I knew my caseworker didn't have my best interest at heart from the beginning, long before pulling me out of college. I was certain of that when she asked me, "Why do you even want to be a writer, Erin?" Do something else with your life…"

I was tired and completely drained when the time came to have another meeting at Penn State Altoona. It was now the middle of 2007 and I hadn't found employment – much less anyone who showed any genuine interest in hiring me. I had a heart full of apprehension and knots in my stomach as I re-entered the same conference room where I was blindsided.

There sat my caseworker, along with a small army of her co-workers. The same staff members on campus who were at the first meeting were also there. I didn't want them to see a repeat of what had already unfolded. My parents were by my side as well, just like they always have been.

I wanted to believe that my caseworker had changed her mind and agree to let me finish what I started three years earlier. I told myself something good had to happen this time around, but hope was stolen from me.

"Erin, I see you don't have a job yet."

"No, ma'am."

"Well, it's been a year."

I swallowed hard as my caseworker dug into me further – saying I would have to settle for an Associate's degree.

Disgusted, my mom looked at me and asked me, "What do you want? Don't look at all these people in this room. Dad and I are proud of you, whether you have a degree or not."

I paused, took a deep breath and said, "I want a Bachelor's degree!"

"This is settled then," my mom declared as she turned to my caseworker. "Erin is re-enrolling here at Penn State Altoona."

That's exactly what I did, despite my caseworker's anger in the conference room was now filled with complete silence. I returned to campus in Fall 2007 with a renewed purpose – and a promise to myself that I wouldn't fall into anyone's trap again. A lot of things were different on a personal level, but I didn't know there was someone who had been waiting to offer me my first job at the local newspaper. Nor was I aware someone else wanted to give me creative control – over the rest of my college career and essentially, my life as a writer.

There will always be naysayers in the crowd. Someone will always try to tear you down. Don't let them. Always go the extra mile. Always reach for the sky and do more than what's expected of you.

Chapter 33

Finding the Strength To Let Go

It's difficult to see where we're going when all we see are roadblocks and obstacles.

It's even more difficult to remember where we've been when something or someone is trying to pull us away from the things we love. The one fact they seem to dismiss, however, is we love those things because we spend so much time building and molding them.

Those who try to tear down what we've built can often distract us. We tend to feel the effects of that distraction long after it comes into our lives, whether it's a simple nudge or a well-calculated punch to the gut. The problem then becomes a matter of holding on for too long and finding the strength to let go.

I never assume things simply happen for the sake of happening. I don't think certain people come into my life at random, either. Everything I've been through is its own story. I could leave it there, but something else has always been attached to the story by the time each is written. So, it made sense when I thought there was a lot more to college than taking a bunch of classes, earning good grades and making a lasting impression.

I was admittedly focused on making an impression on the right people. Up until the end of my sophomore year, there weren't any indications I had made a bad impression on anyone. However, I knew a change had come rather quickly and wasn't handled professionally or gracefully. I also knew whatever happened was going to make me a stronger, more poised human being. What I didn't know was how incredibly influential the last two years of my college career would be – and who was ready and willing to take me under their wing. If anything, I wanted to turn the events of the past year into something positive. I didn't know how I'd do it, but I had faith in myself. It was considerably less than before, but it was good energy regardless. It was energy I needed.

I was sitting in one of my English classes in 2008, knowing I had to be forced to leave campus altogether a year earlier. I still felt betrayed, and I was trying not to let it show. In fact, this was my second chance to prove I shouldn't have been pulled out of my classes at all – much less by my caseworker. None of my professors didn't know what had happened. They just knew I left. That didn't sit well with me, so I continued to do what I've always done – put my head down and work hard.

It was towards the end of my junior year when one of my English professors asked me to stay a few minutes after class. "Sure," I said, not knowing what he was going to say or do. I honestly thought I had written something that wasn't up to par – or perhaps he found out I had been unceremoniously asked to drop out of college.

I didn't jump to any conclusions. I waited a little longer as the room cleared out. My professor pulled out a chair, sat down and made sure everyone had left, before making a simple but very clear observation that would begin to pave the way for my career as a writer.

"Erin," he said in a calm yet excited voice. "I think you should use your disability as a platform for your writing. You're already on to something good with your skill and talent. You need to be utilizing what you have – and doing so in a way that impacts other people."

I couldn't believe it. That was what I'd wanted to do all along! Now, however, there was a sense of affirmation because someone else acknowledged there was a much deeper purpose to my writing. I wasn't waiting for a pat on the back after the debacle with my caseworker, but this was a much-needed boost. It let me know I was still on the right path and people were coming with me this time.

My professor had me pegged in a manner I had never seen or felt before. He knew my strengths, my ambitions, and my goals simply by watching me in his class and reading my work. Not only that, but he had brilliant ideas about how to help me effectively make the most of what I'd been given. It was as if he'd known me my entire life when, in reality, I had only been in his class for a few short months.

This is the same professor who would oversee my senior project at Penn State Altoona a year later– my last opportunity to do something impactful on campus. It would be my chance to leave college the way I wanted to, but it ended up being much more.

You can get through life riding your own waves of positivity. You can succeed. You can even thrive, but you'll be surprised what can happen when someone else believes in you as much as you believe in yourself.

Chapter 34

Bounce Back

Find the moments like a dream. Moments so right, they don't seem real.

We spend so much time navigating through the obstacle course life puts in front of us. We remember how difficult things were – or still are, but don't always embrace our struggles.

We sometimes look at them as a dreaded curse or something was rigged so we would fall flat on our faces. Or maybe someone didn't want us to get as far as they've gotten. There are countless reasons why we stray from our path – whether it's our own doing or a situation that's out of our control. It's only when we take a few steps back we realize how fortunate we truly are.

My senior year at Penn State Altoona was a reminder of all the times I had fallen short – and what I chose to do every time my back was against the wall. I realized why everything I did to get to this point, as well everything I'd do after graduation, had to be so difficult. It wasn't simply because I was used to being knocked down and having to dust myself off. Nor was it because I wanted to be the hero in my own story.

I had to find out what the world truly had to offer me. Most importantly, I had to learn there were other struggles beyond my cerebral palsy. I knew my disability would always be the unavoidable ball and chain attached to me. I also knew it was always going to be its own challenge altogether. I came to terms with that on a much deeper level as my college career was coming to a close.

Now, however, my English professor was not only encouraging me to utilize my disability in a positive way. He was also willing to help me brilliantly put it on display in a full theater production for my senior project – which we would exchange many detailed, thought-provoking e-mails about in the months that followed. Little did I know, he wasn't the only one who wanted to see how bright I could shine.

I made my way down the hall to my next class – a news writing class – after finishing an enlightening conversation with my professor. This particular class was taught by Mr. Ray Eckenrode, the former General Manager of The Altoona Mirror, the local newspaper in Altoona, Pennsylvania. It had been a place where I secretly wanted to work, but I didn't tell anyone because most people thought my passion for writing was a phase that would fade away. I hoped I was making some kind of positive impression in his class, being absolutely certain what I wanted to do with my life. I wasn't prepared for what he would ask me on a chilly night in Fall of 2009.

"So Erin, what's your plan? What do you want to do after you graduate?"

I knew the answer before he even finished asking this question, but patiently waited until he was done talking. If I didn't say anything but the truth now, I thought my chances of realizing a big part of my dream as a writer might be gone.

I wasn't going to experience a moment like this again, so I paused, took a deep breath and said, "I want to work for you!"

"Well, I think we'll be reading a lot more of your work at *The Mirror* sooner than later."

All the while, my mom was listening as this unfolded while she waited to pick me up that night. It was now approximately 9 p.m. and I was exhausted from a full day of classes. I was still sitting in my spot when Mr. Eckenrode walked into the hallway and started talking to my mom.

"I asked Erin what she wants to do after she graduates. She said she wants to work for me," he nervously told her. "Is she serious?"

My mom looked him square in the eye and calmly replied, "Erin isn't kidding. When she puts her mind to something, there's no stopping her. This is the best interview you're going to have right now!"

Mr. Eckenrode was understandably apprehensive about how I'd do this job, instead of doubting my abilities. He approached my longtime adviser for the student newspaper on campus, Margaret Moses, who also worked at The Altoona Mirror at the time. He asked her what I was going to need, thinking he'd have to make major accommodations due to my cerebral palsy.

Margaret smiled and said, "A computer."

That was literally all I needed, along with Margaret's unwavering faith in my ability to write. I was hired as a columnist shortly thereafter, and have been writing for The Mirror ever since. I was still finishing my senior year at Penn State Altoona when I got the news. With my senior project now on the horizon, I had my work cut out for me. but I wouldn't have had it any other way.

You never know when someone is scouting you. Or why they want to pick you out of the crowd. You never know when your next "interview" will be. When that moment arrives, however, be humble and earn respect along the way.

Chapter 35

The Clock Doesn't Stop

The world moves so fast, we often rush through life.

We trick ourselves into thinking we can accomplish more by filling our schedules, skipping three meals a day and forgetting to look at the time.

The one thing we seem to miss during our frenzy, however, is the fact the clock doesn't stop. It doesn't slow down, either. There's no turning the hands back so we can catch up. No wishful thinking. There's only a race to make up for the time we've lost – or the time we have left to do something impactful.

My time as a student at Penn State Altoona was coming to an end. In that time, I laughed, cried, scratched and clawed to get to where I wanted to be, and where I was most comfortable. More importantly, I learned a lot – about myself, my cerebral palsy and how I wanted to move forward after I graduated. I knew writing was going to play a major role in my future – whether or not I had to fight for it.

I had never been as certain about anything else in my life as I was about this. With my new job as a columnist at The

Altoona Mirror secured, I knew I was meant to write for the rest of my life. It had nothing to do with "good timing" or well-placed luck. Nor was this an idea that suddenly popped into my head and resulted in a knee jerk decision to even go to college. I decided to call my column "The View From Here" after tossing around many other possible titles. They all somehow tied in with my cerebral palsy, but sounded far-fetched or forced.

"The View From Here" fit like a glove. I wanted readers to feel as if they were sitting in my chair looking out into the big, vast world right in front of them. All of this was much bigger than any fantasy I could ever dream of. I finally arrived at a place in my life where I knew my disability had a purpose – more important than my own inner struggle with everything surrounding my circumstances.

In fact, it became clear things were slowly falling into place when I saw my name in print, in my local newspaper, for the first time when "The View From Here" debuted during my senior year at Penn State Altoona. Not only that, but I earned nods of approval from my news writing instructors on campus who also worked at The Altoona Mirror. Most importantly, I felt like I was beginning to earn respect as an employee. They not only started to see I took my job seriously, but I think they realized I paid attention to every word I wrote.

It felt surreal to to gain validation from influential people. The message behind my column – it's OK to talk to and interact with me – took a while to catch on with readers. I wasn't shocked or upset, though. I fully expected it, but I also realized something else in the process.

As graduation drew closer, I started to think about what I wanted my senior project to look like. Vivid thoughts of everything I went through to get to this point; the doubt, the pitfalls, and all the times I was told "no" all raced through my mind. Then I thought about the times when I didn't believe or listen to all those negatives.

Where did that take me, and how could I put all of this together in one cohesive package? I had so many ideas, but I wanted to leave my classmates and professors with a feeling of, *Hey, it is OK to talk about disability!* So, I reached out to the same professor who encouraged me to use my disability as a platform for my writing. One e-mail led to another. And another. In about a month, we came up with the idea of having a group of student actors sit in a circle around me on stage.

For my poetry class, I had written enough material that my professor had it made into a booklet. As the actors read each poem, they continued to move in a circle around me. The delayed, almost forced movement represented my everyday struggles while creating the image of a broken down merry-go-round. The finishing touch to this production – the one that meant the most to me – was getting tangled in the pieces of brightly-colored ribbon, which each actor held as they read my poems. The ribbons got tighter and closer to my body each time someone took a turn. It became the physical manifestation of how I often feel about living with a disability.

We rehearsed all of this up until a week or so before the show. My professor and I were confident this was a beautiful way to end my senior year – and the right way to say goodbye. However, I wasn't prepared for the flood of emotion.

Some things are good. Others might be great, but it's what you make out of them that truly matters.

Chapter 36

Represent Yourself and Let It Out

Why do we hold onto things we know will fade away?

It's easy to take things for granted. It's even easier to a meticulous painting or a clear blue sky and think its beauty is temporary. We tell ourselves it won't last. Or it won't mean as much years from now.

The question becomes, 'Why do we hold onto things we know will fade away?' It's likely to cause pain and anguish if we get too close or become attached. Yet, we run the risk of missing out on so much if we don't make some sort of connection. That beautiful sky, painting or whatever we're looking at, might lose its importance to us. It might turn into another object or fixture in the world if we don't look at it in the right light.

I've never wanted that to be the case with many things in my life. I didn't want to get into the habit of thinking my circumstances make everything dark and dreary. I've never wanted anyone around me to feel that way, either – especially the people who were in the audience during my senior project at Penn State Altoona.

It was a bitterly cold night in December 2009 as people began to pile into a large room on campus. I greeted everyone with a smile and thanked them for coming. I couldn't help but glance over at the stage where I'd hopefully be giving those in attendance something to remember, but also saying goodbye to my professors and peers at the same time.

I didn't make any promises that the audience was going to see a great show, but I was given an amazing opportunity to bring my emotions to life in a way I never thought possible. My English professor who oversaw the production spotted me and walked over to check on things before I went on stage.

"How are you feeling now?" he asked, knowing I'd been nervous from working relentlessly on this – and rehearsing with the student actors whom we had chosen.

"I'm still a little shaky," I admitted. "I'm ready, though!"

"Great!" he said. "You made this happen, Erin. This is your story, and we're here to help you tell it in a new way.

I'm excited for people to see you tonight!"

I wasn't about to let this pass me by, now everything had come together and was actually happening. It was bittersweet too, because I knew this would be one of the few times – maybe the only time – when most of the people who took a chance on me during my college career would be gathered in one room. The fact that I had never been in a theater production before, much less directed one, made this even more exhilarating.

I didn't want to let them down. More importantly, I didn't want the people involved in this production to feel like they wasted their time. I couldn't worry about any of that now.

It was show time. I took a deep breath before lining my wheelchair up with the makeshift ramp to the stage. My professor followed and gave a brief but beautiful introduction. When everyone was settled, the poetry I had written suddenly came to life – and the audience was with me every step of the way.

They heard every word of every poem. They saw the stiff, rough movement as my student maneuvered around me in a circle as they read. I looked out into the audience and saw people crying and wiping tears from their eyes without saying a word. I was tangled in a web of colorful ribbon about two hours later, feeling like I had done more than simply say goodbye to so many people who impacted my life up until this point.

For the first time in a long time, I didn't have to explain why I'm in a wheelchair or why my legs don't work. I didn't have to pretend having a disability is a simple matter of getting through each day. Every person in the room connected with what was happening on stage in some way. it wasn't just a look that said, "Wow, this is good!" I think it was a combination of gratitude and a genuine appreciation for a glimpse into what my life is really like when I struggle.

It felt liberating to be able to represent myself. I still feel that way every time I write. I hope it never goes away because it's a huge part of why I started my journey as a writer in the first place.

When the feeling creeps in, don't push it down into your gut. Let it out and express it. It might be scary, but this is what propels to you things you'd never imagine.

Chapter 37

Accomplishment on Your Own Terms

Rising to the occasion when no one expects it.

The feeling of accomplishment is beautiful. It takes us to a place that once seemed so far away. a place where no one expected us to go, or even dream of going. When we finally get there, however, it's often a different experience altogether.

The people who doubted us become silent and those who have stuck with us proudly shout our praises from the rooftops. Our crowd then gets divided into two groups. We start to see who was truly by our side all along, but what happens when we've done everything we set out to do?

Where do we go when we've reached the top of the mountain in front of us? Most importantly, who's still going to be there when we make our next move?

December 2009. My second graduation from Penn State Altoona had finally arrived. It wasn't what I originally planned for. Nor was it what some people expected me to go through with, especially after my caseworker forced me to drop out two years earlier.

I wanted to forget my first gradation even took place, but I reminded myself it happened this way for a reason. Or else I wouldn't have had the opportunities the campus afforded me to grow, try new things and find out who I was.

The moment stolen from me was about to come full circle – as was everything else that made this day so emotional. It was stronger than the sense of knowing I could move on with my life. It was even bigger than knowing I now had free reign to truly start my career. This was about the notion of looking out into the audience and seeing an empty seat.

I never forgot how I had lost my grandfather the year before my high school graduation. I didn't forget how tightly my family held me when I came home from school to find out he had suffered a massive heart attack. I thought about him every day as I was jumping through every hoop to get where I wanted to be in life. Now, he wasn't here to see where I ended up. Or to see I was on my way to becoming "the best writer in the world", as he always said I'd be – even before I had garnered any success.

I looked up to see my family in the crowd as I waited to be introduced with the rest of my graduating class. My nana, who had had knee surgery, was in considerable pain but smiled from ear-to-ear. I saw her glance up at the lights to reassure me I didn't make it this far on my own. At that moment, every memory I ever had came rushing back so quickly and vividly.

There were other things that happened along the way, which I kept relatively quiet about. Things such as getting fitted for a new wheelchair every five years or celebrating my

21st birthday at Red Lobster with a strawberry margarita. I somehow deemed these moments as typical and normal. They always stuck out in my memory, but I didn't think they needed to be singled out. Those moments were special because they reminded me of a short time in my life when almost everything was simple.

They're still meaningful because I can vividly remember how they made me feel. The immediate impact of my grandfather's death, however, carried a weight that has never gotten easier to bear. That, combined with the butterflies in my stomach, made graduating college this second time around even more bittersweet than it already was.

I was about to close a very important chapter in my life – perhaps one in which I never would've had the chance to write if I hadn't done what I did. I knew in my heart this part of my story couldn't have unfolded any other way. I had to question a lot of things. Most importantly, however, I had to prove my cerebral palsy wasn't the center of my universe.

I wanted to accomplish as much as I could on my own terms. That's all I've ever wanted to do, but two fancy pieces of paper from my college didn't validate it. My determination did.

Material things are great. They might fill a void and make you happy, but they don't equal success. They're not always going to be there for you, either. Only the people who matter will stay true. That should be reason enough to rise to the occasion – not when we're asked to do so, but especially when no one expects it.

Chapter 38

What Paths Life Takes

Make it happen, let it happen, or somewhere in the middle?

Everyone has their own opinions about how life is supposed to unfold. Some say whatever is meant to be, will be. Others say we have to have a plan before we can chase our dreams.

Then there are those who simply take things as they come. If there's a plan, that's great. If there isn't, they make it up as they go along. There's no real direction, but there isn't a lack of ambition, either.

Where do we fall on the delicate line between those who go after what they want and those who let things happen? How do we know if we're being too passive or too headstrong? More importantly, what happens when we start to think there's only one way to get to the pot of gold at the end of the rainbow?

I didn't have a blueprint. There wasn't a master plan, except to write – and keep writing, no matter what happened after I graduated from college. It wasn't a promise I made to myself. Nor was it one I had been held to. It was, however, a feeling that never faded. The fire kept burning bright, even though there were some people who tried to put it out.

The flames of determination and desire rose so high inside of me I couldn't ignore them anymore. I never pushed them to the side, but they did, however, become part of a much bigger picture. I finally knew what to do with everything I'd learned in life so far – and now had the resources I needed, but I waited to see if the right opportunities came along. And they did.

I began to receive offers to write for small publications, within roughly six months after graduating from Penn State Altoona on my own terms. I was surprised but very humbled at the same time. I didn't have much to show for myself in terms of compelling articles or noteworthy accomplishments in the writing industry. The only thing I had was my small column in The Altoona Mirror – which had only been running for a few short months. In that time, my work had garnered the respect of my local community and people started to look forward to reading one article every month.

This was no longer about my cerebral palsy. I didn't have to write simply to prove myself anymore – at least not to anyone in my hometown who read my column. I could write because I loved doing it – a privilege which I felt I earned. I wanted to eventually reach a broader audience, but in this moment, I just wanted to take in the fact I was writing on a monthly basis. Little did I know, everything I wanted as a writer, journalist, and poet was going to come to me in waves.

In 2010, I began the editing process for *To Cope and To Prevail,* the autobiography of Dr. Ilse-Rose Warg, my former German professor at Penn State Altoona. I had never edited a book before, nor did I know how to read anything written in another language. I wasn't particularly looking for an editing project, either.

I knew I had to help when she told me she was working on the book for many years, but it fell by the wayside because she didn't have an Editor. I could tell her hopes of finishing and publishing the book were deflated, with every word of broken English she spoke.

The agreement to embark on such a huge undertaking started a year earlier, when I took a class she designed to teach me how to read German, to ensure I had enough foreign language credits to graduate. Ironically, Dr. Warg noticed my passion for writing, as well as my willingness to learn.

"You put words together very well, Erin," she said before asking if I would be interested in editing her book.

"Oh, thank you," I replied innocently.

I had no idea how long the book was, but I was confident in my skill and knowledge of English grammar and syntax. I agreed to step in as her Editor, not knowing she was writing the book in English – as well as in German. I paused and asked myself, "How am I going to do this?"

It was the same question I had asked myself countless times, but I had an answer now. Two years, many grueling hours and almost 300 pages later, the book was finished and available for the world to read. Having my name listed in the book as Editor was an accomplishment I didn't expect, which made the project even more meaningful. I saw my professor as just that – a teacher – before coming onboard to do this. Now, I see her as someone who endured a tremendous amount of pain, sacrifice and struggle to build the life she once could only dream of.

Taking this project on at this particular point in my career was admittedly the biggest challenge for me as a budding writer. The fact it happened right after college didn't make it any easier, but it prepared me for the relentless daily pace that comes with my line of work. It also made me a better writer and human being. For that, I'll never be able to repay Dr. Warg.

You can tell yourself there's only one way to do something. You can travel that path for a while, too. When something risky comes along, however, don't turn away until you see the impact it can have. You might be missing out on the best thing in your life.

Chapter 39

The Lies in Our Goodbyes

The loss of a loved one is never easy, but saying goodbye can become an opportunity.

There are times when we look at ourselves and think we're not good enough. We tell ourselves an overused lie "we can't do this or that for whatever reason – and say the stone we left unturned is safer the way it is." Or, "it's best to let someone else take the risk of turning the stone over."

We turn away, lost and deflated. Then, there's a moment when we look in the mirror and see a reflection of our heroes. They're always the ones who don't wear capes, but they do something at some point and we say, "I wish I could be like them!" or "Hey, I can do what they're doing!"

I've never wanted to be a carbon copy of anyone else. Nor have I wanted to ride someone's coattails. I've always just wanted to be myself – regardless of how difficult my journey was going to be. Or how much it changed me. With the long, meticulous editing process for Dr. Warg's memoir finished and more offers for work in addition to my column in The Altoona Mirror, writing was quickly becoming much more than my chosen profession. It was a way for me to keep the personal burdens of my disability at bay.

They stayed with me as I adjusted to adulthood, like children who grow up too fast, but who never leave home. I started thinking about what my life would be like if I didn't have the friends and family I had. My two grandmothers, one on each side of my parents' families, were the only grandparents I had who were still alive. . Both were proud of my accomplishments in writing and graduating from college, but they had very contrasting ways of showing it.

It was the beginning of 2012 by now and my nana – my grandfather's widow – was preparing for heart surgery. Her doctor found a valve leaking around her heart during a routine check-up. The valve went undetected for months and caused her chest pain.

It was determined she needed surgery to replace the leaking valve and relieve the pressure around her heart. The procedure was deemed high risk because of her age. Being the strong woman she was, my nana agreed to have this done. She was feeling good up until a few months before. It was early February when she said she had to have the operation because she wanted to spend more time with her grandchildren.

Two months later, in late April, she was gone. The surgery was successful, but immediate complications kept mounting. Doctors sent her from one hospital to another, draining fluid from her body and inserting tubes into her skin to try to save her. No one believed she was the healthy, vivacious Bingo player my family said she was, because she had gone through so much by the time she arrived at each hospital.

All the doctors could see was a frail, old shell of a woman confined to a bed. She was a patient with a number. My family stayed by her side through it all, but it was clear her time with us was fading.

She quietly passed away in a nursing home in Ebensburg, Pennsylvania – after a long and painful fight. She had been hooked up to a ventilator and could no longer speak. She could only nod her head. My mom and uncle, two of her three children, were the first ones called in to make the final decision for doctors to remove all the tubes – and say goodbye.

I can't speak for my family on this, but I can remember my heart shattering like a piece of precious glass when I heard my nana had passed. It got to the point where we all knew her death was a matter of time. Something inside me told me she knew, too.

I also considered what would have happened if I didn't fight for my dream of being a writer. The only time I could find any middle ground, however, was when I was by myself and typing on my computer.

It all somehow intertwined with the notion of how I'd react if I lost everything, and thinking about what I already lost – probably too much. It wasn't because I was afraid or anxious. It was instead because I now had one grandparent who was still alive. I knew I'd eventually lose her too. I just hoped it wasn't as terrifying.

In the months following my nana's passing, writing became my escape. I wasn't worried about getting hired anywhere or making a name for myself. I simply wanted to write because it made me feel human and my pain didn't seem so unbearable. I wasn't ready to shine again. Nor was I prepared to tell myself another hard truth, but I would soon get an unexpected opportunity to build myself back up. And do so in a big way.

When the world seems scary, face it. Be honest. You might uncover something that has been there all along.

Chapter 40

Vulnerability Is a Scary Kind of Magic

You never know who might be out there watching and waiting with an opportunity.

Life can become a big, predictable cycle of repetition. We often get into a routine, follow it until it feels right, and tend to not stray from it. The comfort of knowing we'll wake up and do the same things every day turns into an unspoken promise.

It doesn't matter if it's good or bad for us. At least not when it feels good. We fall so far down the hole created by our own comfort we don't want to dig ourselves out. There comes a moment, however, when we realize we can't stay in the hole. We're forced to ask ourselves, 'Was I wrong to allow myself to get too comfortable?'

This question raced through my mind after my nana's passing in early 2012. I became so comfortable with my life the way it was. My column in The Altoona Mirror was gaining more readership each month it was being published as I continued to receive offers to write for small publications. It was a slow start, but I welcomed it because this was exactly what I wanted all along. More importantly, it was what I had worked for since the moment I learned how to put words together. I didn't want anything to jeopardize that.

I pushed the thought of things changing to the side. I thought losing someone, particularly my grandparents, was years – maybe decades away. It hadn't occurred to me I didn't need to be a certain age to not only witness death, but to also say goodbye, until it happened. My grandfather's death came very unexpectedly, but I was 17 years old when he passed. I was practically a baby in an adult's world.

I wasn't ready to let go then, and I still didn't want to tell myself the truth now. It became abundantly clear my nana wasn't going to be with my family much longer. She had suffered from so many complications following her heart surgery that a goodbye became expected, and the best thing for her.

I was left to look inside myself and admit I was being selfish. I believed the delusional lie that things last forever – at least when it came to the people whom I hold dear. In the back of my mind, however, it wasn't a matter of delusion at all. It was more about realizing what was right in front of me.

I also wrestled with the fact I now had one grandmother left on my dad's side of the family. She had never been in good health, and she never truly looked passed my cerebral palsy – not nearly as much as she had convinced herself she did. At this point, I was writing enough to keep my column going and my mind in a good place. I wasn't looking to overwhelm myself with work. I didn't want to become lazy and complacent, either. My family unfortunately had only a few years left with my grandmother, as she, too, passed away after my nana's death.

The immediate impact of everything going on around me radiated through my body. I started to think it was all too much. Perhaps too heavy to bear. I realized I need something to break this cycle – this sad, unwelcome state of mind.

Before October 28, 2012, editing Dr. Warg's memoir was the only big milestone in my career worth mentioning. I hadn't written anything on a national level. Everything I knew about taking a risk at this point — as well as the absolute fear and hesitation that comes with it — had to do with my cerebral palsy. It wasn't because I didn't know any better. It was because I felt my disability was no longer the only thing that truly presented a challenge.

However, something felt different on this cold October night – a feeling to make the blood in my fingertips flow. I cautiously but rather intriguingly read through an e-mail from one Cameron Conaway.

My first thought was, *Who's Cameron Conaway?*

I'd never heard of him before, nor did I know what he was about and what his story was. I'd only seen a few pictures of whom I assumed was him on Facebook. Moreover, I was confused as to why he was reaching out to me. What could I possibly have to offer a complete stranger — much less a stranger who started out as an MMA fighter and was now Social Justice Editor of The Good Men Project, an online publication I'd never heard of?

I carefully read through some more general information he included in the e-mail. I was utterly and completely blown away as I went down the list of his accolades — accomplished poet, writer — earning him the distinction of being known as The Warrior Poet around the world — and a prominent voice against human trafficking — but that still didn't explain why he was making an effort to connect with me.

Then, as if it were a beam of light in the darkness, my eyes gravitated towards this:

> "I read your work in The [Altoona] Mirror. I truly believe you have the potential to be one of the leading disability writers in the country, if not THE top disability writer. Would you be interested in writing a piece for the Social Justice section of The Good Men Project?"

I sat at my computer in silence for a moment. I stared at those words until my eyes stung. It was if I'd been injected with some type of undiscovered antibody or kryptonite. I knew Cameron understood and could truly grasp the one thing that's taken the rest of the world an eternity to grasp: there's more to me than just my disability. He didn't see my cerebral palsy as a reason to sweep certain topics under the rug.

Cameron asked me to write more articles in the following months. I wrote each one with the intention of showing him he didn't make the wrong decision in offering me a job. In doing so, I began to gain a new following with a new audience on a national basis. It felt liberating to continue to chip away at a very high glass ceiling, but nothing was more satisfying than knowing someone was watching – and waiting for the right moment to reach out.

Vulnerability can be scary. It puts unbelievable weight on your shoulders and makes you take steps into the unknown – but that's where the real magic is.

Chapter 41

When the Stars Align, or Don't

There is no wrong turn to the promised land.

There comes a time in life when we have a clear idea of where we're going and what we want. We might have started down the path we thought was going to lead us to The Promised Land. We might even think our current situation – whatever it might be – is as good as it's going to get.

When we stop and look around, however, we see there's more work to be done. Obtaining the things we truly want always takes more blood, sweat, and tears than we initially anticipate. We may travel other roads on our way to doing so – not because it's necessarily the best path to take. Nor because we've been advised to go that way.

Sometimes we have to pass by dark places on the way to getting what we want. As I would find out, though, we don't have to stay there.

I was at a strange place in my life by the end of 2012. I had everything I wanted as I was building my career, but I was empty and broken inside. The voices who once bellowed, "My granddaughter is the best writer in the world!" were gone, I had to push the sense of loss down into the pit of my stomach while I watched my readership at The Good Men Project grow. I was now in a position where my work was being read by everyone made me feel I was doing something right.

My work was no longer just for me, or the locals who read my column in Altoona. It was now accessible to anyone who took the time to read it. Most importantly, I tried to write from a genuinely inclusive perspective – which developed naturally. I think Cameron saw in my writing something he felt was missing at The Good Men Project.

I was motivated to keep the momentum with a feeling of immense gratitude. He had hired me on no other basis except for the quality of my work. I got the feeling Cameron knew I wasn't trying to be something I wasn't. He knew I wouldn't randomly put an article together simply because I was happy to finally be writing on a national level.

I think Cameron knew the quality of my work matched my integrity with every article I wrote. I wasn't going to give him anything less than my best, and he didn't expect anything less in return. This was a beautiful, important moment because no one truly expected anything from me. Anyone who crossed paths with me up until this point knew I gave my heart and soul every time I set my mind on doing something.

People knew I was going to finish whatever I started, but the certainty always came with some degree of convincing on my part. Not with Cameron and the rest of the editorial staff at The Good Men Project. It felt great knowing there was a group of people out there who believed in my work as much as I did. Having Cameron as my Editor helped me tremendously because he was open to any ideas I had, and constantly offered his own ideas about how to expand on them. He had confidence in my work and allowed me the freedom to do my own 'thing'.

The overwhelming sense I had to live the best life I could possibly live rushed me. It wasn't because I felt old or thought I should have been doing something else other than writing. It was rather because I knew I could comfortably put my cerebral palsy to the side without feeling guilty or ashamed.

I wasn't going to forget about it or ignore it. Nor was I going to pretend that being a writer with a disability automatically gave me a pass to say what I wanted, however I wanted to say it. Getting hired at my first national writing job – much less getting hired anywhere – wasn't about having the opportunity to ramble on about how difficult my life is. Or to give readers a reason to feel bad for me. I understood <u>The Good Men Project</u> was a platform with a diverse blend of opinions and perspectives. If I was going to continue to add mine, I'd have to make smart choices.

I had to learn how to effectively weave my disability into my writing. It was an extremely valuable lesson I don't think I could have learned anywhere else, in any other way. It felt like the more I wrote, the more preparation I had for the next opportunity to come my way. Little did I know. the next thing that happened would be one of the biggest steps in my life.

One thing always leads to another. You may not realize it at first, but you'll know when the stars begin to align. When they don't align, question it, smile, and know it happened. Most importantly though, simply be grateful.

Chapter 42

What's Worthwhile to You?

Complexity, simplicity, and doing a good thing.

We all want life to be simple. We want certain things to come more easily than others, but sometimes we don't know a good thing when we see it. Or we have too much of a good thing, and end up wasting it trying to figure out if it's actually beneficial to us.

We can regard life as something to teach us a lesson. We might even think of it as an opportunity to find the best parts of ourselves. With that comes a responsibility to recognize what we can do for other people while sharing the best parts of who we are.

By the beginning of 2013, I started to get the sense that my writing wasn't just doing something for me anymore. I could tell it was doing something good for those who read it, as people were e-mailing me with comments equally as thoughtful as powerful. I was simply grateful I was able to write so freely – and do so with Cameron's expertise and guidance.

I was balancing my time between The Altoona Mirror and The Good Men Project, making sure everything I wrote was up to par. I slowly weaved things I learned from Cameron into my column for *The Mirror* – and vice-versa. It was a chance to bring two parts of my world together. Most importantly, it was something I wouldn't have known how to do if I hadn't built a solid foundation early on in my career.

I learned very quickly that predicting how others respond to what's put in front of them is nearly impossible, especially if it's in the public eye. I also understood it wasn't my job to tell people what to think, but I still had a responsibility to give them something to think about. I wrote my articles with that in mind – and it clicked. People began to connect with my work in their own ways, and it sparked a feeling of personal pride in me.

I wasn't writing about world problems or how to solve them. Nor was I trying to change their minds about anything in particular. I was simply sharing my experiences living with cerebral palsy, and researching disability-related issues to write about.

My writing and topics were enough for people to not only keep reading, but to also look forward to when my articles were published. I knew my initial goal of helping others feel comfortable talking and interacting with me was starting to come full circle. The decision to fully incorporate my disability into my writing, however, was a tough one.

I was skeptical because my circumstances are very personal to me. I keep them close to my heart for that reason – and because they're not things I have the luxury of forgetting about. I knew cerebral palsy is one of the most common disabilities out there, but like everything else in the world, not everyone reacts the same way to the stigma attached to having a disability. I also thought about vulnerability becoming a factor if I put myself on display. Or even parts of myself.

I was already vulnerable by default. The questions then became, *'Should I risk making myself even more vulnerable by telling my story?'* and *'Would that make me brave – or just foolish?'* The last thing to cross my mind was my effort to make my writing public. I spent so much time trying to figure out what I'd do if my work was ever read by anyone outside of my family and friends. What would happen if someone didn't agree with something I wrote?

I was in a position where I could now find these things out for myself, and had gained a decent following on a local basis with my column in The Altoona Mirror, which seemed to be growing. Now, however, I'd been writing for The Good Men Project long enough for readers to follow my work there as well.

This was completely surreal because these were people who I didn't even know. Not only that, but they weren't from my small town of Altoona, Pennsylvania and most likely never read my column in The Altoona Mirror. The deeper I delved into the subject of disability, the more appreciation people showed for my work.

In a moment of honesty, I realized I didn't plan for any of this. The plan was to tell my story if I ever got the opportunity to do so. I didn't have a blueprint for what happens when I'm praised for something I love to do. I did know by now, however, I wanted to bring everyone with me on this part of my journey – regardless of whether they had a disability or not.

You might not have a lot in your pocket. You might not be powerful or famous, but it's important to set your mind on doing something worthwhile. When you set out to do it, make sure to bring as many people as possible along for the ride.

Chapter 43

Respect Rolls the Dice

Will they believe enough to gamble on you?

It's often difficult to know what someone else is thinking. It's even more difficult to understand why they do the things they do. Or why they decide to take a chance on something not set in stone.

Sometimes it's none of our business. It may not be our place to question other people's choices or motives. There are certain times, however, when those things do become a part of our lives. Not because we've pushed the other person to the point where they feel uncomfortable. Nor because we want something from them. Perhaps it's because they have our best interest at heart and want to see us succeed.

The very first time I put pen to paper, it wasn't to achieve a goal. It wasn't to write the next Great American Classic. It was, however, what I believed to be my salvation. I've always kept that in mind, but it wasn't simply a thought anymore. It became my foundation as I made my way through 2013. I was writing new material on a steady basis and things were finally falling into place.

I was writing so much, it didn't feel like work. It was so natural, but part of it still felt like a wildly surreal dream. I thought this "dream" couldn't get any better. Little did I know, however, my career was about to get another unexpected boost.

I was working on an article for The Good Men Project when Cameron e-mailed me with an idea that seemed so far away at the time.

> "Hey Erin," he wrote. "Have you ever considered writing a trial article for The Huffington Post?"

I began my reply with, "Yes, I have thought about it…"

At this point, I was confident enough in my ability to write to take chances. I understood why I needed to take calculated risks if I wanted others in the writing industry to take me seriously. I also felt my decision to weave my cerebral palsy into my work might be an asset if I were to have something published by The Huffington Post. The thought of being published by such a prestigious publication was significant; I had always wanted to write for them. It was something, however, I thought should happen later in my career – when I had more time to prepare.

I expressed this to Cameron, and how important this was to me. I didn't want to write an article simply for the sake of having my name in the public eye even more than it already was. I was well aware of the prestige attached to Huffington, having read many of their stories over the years. If I was going to do this, I was going to give it my all. And then some.

Cameron responded very confidently yet calmly, saying, "I think you're ready now, Erin." It was as if he knew what I was capable of before I knew, and I'm forever grateful. I also think he could sense I handled every opportunity I received with professionalism and pride, whether it was large or small.

Knowing that he had that much faith in my ability to write, at such an early stage in my career, made me feel like I was doing something that was bigger than myself. I did what I did because I wanted to do it – not because people were starting to know who I was.

I wanted more. The magic in my fingers began to truly bleed out. I let it flow until my hesitation was gone — until all I was left with were words. They inadvertently paved a path to a career and helped me find my real voice that rings loud and clear today – all the way to The Huffington Post and beyond. Writing for Huffington allowed me the opportunity to connect with other writers from all over the world.

In my hometown of Altoona, PA, I've affectionately become known as "the girl who writes for The Altoona Mirror." It's a distinction I'm still trying to wrap my head around for so many years. Now, however, I want to continue to grow and do what I can to change the perception of disability.

I feel it's a responsibility built into my job as a writer. Most importantly, it's a constant reminder that respect is not given, it's earned. When that happens, the sky is truly the limit.

Chapter 44

Be the Moment

Sometimes, you have to let another person take the wheel.

We all wonder if we're doing enough sometimes. We often watch the foundation of humanity fall apart because the world can be an unfair place. The feeling of helplessness creeps in and we're left to wonder what we could, or should, have done.

There are other times, however, when we fall short on a personal level. We have to ask ourselves, *Have I done everything I can to help myself and others? Am I prepared to work hard when I don't feel like working – or when it seems like everyone else is sitting and watching?*

Perhaps it's a simple question like, *Am I happy?* or *Do I have everything I truly want in life?*

I was fortunate to be able to answer these questions without the feeling of overwhelming doubt going into 2014.

I was confident my work was doing something worthwhile – not only for myself, but for others as well. I also felt like the stigma and pressure easier to deal with. of having a disability became easier to deal with. I still had to prove myself, but now, it was because I was chipping away at an extremely high glass ceiling in the writing industry.

Having cerebral palsy only made the task more difficult, as it has been since the day my career started. The final months of 2013, however, proved to be an entirely different kind of pressure as I began writing the first draft of my first article for The Huffington Post. it wasn't simply an article I had wanted to write for a long time. Nor was it something I'd been procrastinating over on purpose.

The premise of the article – how my cerebral palsy doesn't define my life – was well-received by the handful of people whom I quietly told the idea to. They were established writers – most of whom I crossed paths with at Penn State Altoona during my time there as a student. Not only that, but Cameron was always within reach since hiring me at The Good Men Project in 2012.

I knew it would be a huge step for my career if I did this right. However, there was also a very high possibility the article would be rejected – as rejection is a big part of any routine as a writer. I told myself I could resubmit the article to the Editors at Huffington if it didn't get published on my first attempt. I understood that was and always will be the tough nature of the writing industry, but I had a different way of thinking this time.

I asked myself, *How long have I been waiting and preparing for this moment?* Then, I proceeded to tell myself I might not be as prepared for this in six months, as I was right then. I needed to write this article and try to get it in front of

Huffington's editors. It didn't matter if I could resubmit it in a week or six months. If I wasn't ready at this very moment, I might have waited and essentially missed out on what I then regarded as the biggest opportunity of my life.

All of this writing, drafting and pondering led up to January 2014. My article was finished. I didn't want to tinker with it any more than I had in the past month, for fear I'd lose its integrity. I reached out to Cameron to let him know I was finally ready to send my work to The Huffington Post for review. Having articles published there before, Cameron allowed me to send mine to him to give one final read through.

"I think you're golden, Erin," he said. "Do you feel comfortable with what you wrote?"

"Yes," I replied. "I'm ready for this!"

With that, the waiting game began. And so did the pressure. It started to mount as I tried to send my work to as many publications as I could. Submitting my work to different places has always been a part of my routine as a writer, but it helped to pass the time while I waited to hear about my article. I looked at it as a welcomed distraction, which again didn't feel much like work.

It felt good to be able to get to a point where I could simply enjoy what I was doing. I still had deadlines to meet, but I didn't feel rushed. I found time to just live my life as a writer. It wasn't a goal or something I had been thinking about. It happened naturally and it was a beautiful thing.

I did not want it to end. Nor did I want the feeling attached to it to go away – and it didn't. After a few nail-biting weeks of waiting, I received word my article had been accepted for publication at The Huffington Post – the place I'd only read about since I was a little girl.

Sometimes you need to stop. You need to breathe and take everything in, instead of trying to be in the driver's seat all the time. It's the best medicine, next to laughter. It helps you focus. Most importantly, it helps you appreciate the world around you.

Chapter 45

The Fine Line Between Integrity and Self-Care

Sometimes, the cost of success means separating the personal from the professional.

There are certain things in life we shouldn't question. Some of those things are obvious, like the sky is above us and the sun is our star. We don't debate these things because it's been etched into our brain as fact – we can know it for ourselves.

Then, there are things we don't have to question. They might not be apparent to other people, but we know how vital they are to our own well-being. Sometimes that's all it takes – being fully aware of what we hold dear and doing everything we can to protect it.

There are also certain things we choose to share with others.

At some point, however, there has to be a line between public and private territory. The question is, where do we draw that line?

These questions came with an incredible amount of responsibility. I put a lot of pressure on myself because my cerebral palsy had become the driving force behind my work – and I welcomed that. I finally understood how to utilize my circumstances as a way to help others, and it felt surreal.

I had made a conscious decision to put my disability on display, which meant putting myself in the public eye. No one else could have made that choice for me. I knew exactly why my cerebral palsy had to be a part of my career if I wanted my writing to continue to have an impact. All of this was accompanied by a sense I had arrived at a comfortable, almost peaceful place in my life.

I wasn't willing to jeopardize the peace. If anything, I wanted to preserve and savor it because it didn't come easily. I had a feeling it would only become more difficult to keep peace at the center of my life as my career blossomed – and I wanted to be as prepared as I could be.

A few weeks into January 2014, my first article for The Huffington Post was published. Chills ran down my spine as my name, followed by my own words, were printed in a major publication. Comments and support began pouring in from my family, friends, and faithful readers. I knew my grandparents were looking down on me from afar, with the biggest smiles on their faces. With this joy, however, came a very genuine reminder: I needed to make another important decision.

Outside of my work, I was hesitant to share certain things with the public. I was trying to balance the business of life – being a good daughter, sister, and niece while still being a good writer. I had to choose what I wanted the world to know, and what I wanted to keep to myself. It seemed like an easy thing to do, but I quickly found out that could not have been farther from the truth.

Many of my friends had fallen on hard times, trying to fight battles they didn't ask to be in and heal old wounds, as well as new ones. These were the same friends who I had met in college. When I met them, I had no right to claim life was unfair or my circumstances were too heavy. I still didn't have that right, even if it was now years after the fact.

Had I not stopped and listened to their stories, I might have never learned about the depth of the human soul. Nor would I have known what true inspiration is. I made a promise to myself to make every effort to be there for them, and be their safety net like they've been for me countless times.

There was a long stretch of days where I wanted to burst into tears because I was at a painful crossroad. I didn't want to hurt my friends by sharing what was happening, but I was in agony by remaining silent. I knew I couldn't break down because I still had responsibilities – to my family, my employers and most importantly, my friends.

They were going through situations I couldn't even fathom. Not only did I make a promise to listen, but I also made a promise to keep my integrity intact. I had to choose between my personal life and losing very close, dear friends. It got to the point where the right choice was so obvious I couldn't ignore it. Nor did I want to.

At this very moment, I decided to draw a line personally and professionally. It was a line I never planned to draw. It became one, however, I needed to draw, right then and there. I didn't want to be the reason for anyone's pain. I wanted, more than anything else, to stay in the public eye so I could continue to serve a purpose.

Some things must be set aside for you – and only you. It might not be easy. Chances are, it won't even be what everyone around you wants. You have to take care of yourself at some point. If you don't, how can you expect to do the same for anyone else when they need you the most?

Chapter 46

Appreciate the Process

It's easy to get lost in the hustle and bustle of life, so lost we often take things for granted.

It takes little effort to look at someone of high stature and think, *Wow, they have it easy!* or *They have it all!* We might see the fancy cars and the material gains of their success. The part we tend to overlook, however, is what they went through to put themselves in that position. Most importantly, we can become envious. Then, we think about the things we don't have – or tease ourselves while looking at everything money can buy.

No one truly knew who I was before I started to write. No one knew what was underneath the veil of my cerebral palsy – and many people didn't take the time to look. In fact, there were times when I thought writing was one of the few things to help me feel normal. It would be foolish to try to convince myself or anyone else I still don't feel that way sometimes.

It became obvious to me writing is a lonely profession, as one of my English professors at Penn State Altoona called it. I didn't have any friends who were writers years ago when I decided I wanted to do this for the rest of life.

My list of things I need has grown since, even though writer friends are still hard to come by.

I also found out rather quickly there are no shortcuts or handouts in this line of work, which fit my lifestyle perfectly. There was also a lot of rejection – from editors, publishers, and others within the writing industry. I began to think it was because I was writing about disability on a deeper, larger scale, but again quickly learned about the very big role rejection plays in being a writer.

As I submitted my work to various publications, including book publishers, I started spending eight hours a day on my computer. It ended up being the equivalent of a full-time job – considering the fact that it takes double the time and energy for me to get things done due to my cerebral palsy.

Nonetheless, I kept my pace heading into the end of 2014. I was writing for The Good Men Project as well The Huffington Post while still staying on track with my local column for The Altoona Mirror. I've always felt as if each publication that I've been fortunate enough to write for, prepared me for whatever came next. Now, it wasn't simply in my head. I was seeing proof that everything I did or wrote was a stepping stone to something bigger.

It got to the point where I actually had a schedule to follow and commitments to keep. One of the biggest things I wanted now, was for those who read my work to know that being a writer is always a process and a tedious one, at that. My friends and family were well aware I was aiming to get my career where I wanted it to be, but I sometimes felt like they were the only ones who truly understood why I gave up so much of my free time.

I also wanted people to realize I wasn't going away. I wasn't going to stop writing, even if no one was reading what I wrote because I still wanted to help someone by telling my stories. Most importantly, I hoped readers understood I didn't become a writer for fame or fortune. Nor because it was seemingly the only job I was qualified for. I stuck with it because I simply love to write.

All of this is still important to me. It's still the backbone of why I do what I do. If anything, I hope others recognize and appreciate it as much as I do. Things began to shift as my readership grew on a local and national basis. The more work I put out into the world, the more it seemed like readers understood where I was coming from as a writer. More importantly, it felt like they not only embraced me but also accepted my perspective.

That didn't happen overnight. Neither did my ability to live the life of a writer. There was the writing aspect – the most obvious part. Then, there was the responsibility of not only finding a routine but also sticking to it as more deadlines came my way. Readers started to catch on to the fact I wasn't just sitting at my computer and writing random words. I was researching, checking my facts and doing whatever needed to be done before anything with my name on it got accepted for publication.

It was now October 2014. I was working on an article fairly late at night when I received an e-mail. Cameron, who had served as Social Justice Editor at <u>The Good Men Project</u> upon hiring me, decided to step down and move forward with his career. I was shocked because Cameron is one of the most dedicated people I've had the privilege of working for. I took a deep breath, trying to process this overwhelming news. Just as I came back to reality, I read this line in the e-mail:

"We are looking for someone to fill Cameron's position."

I lost my breath for a moment. I immediately wanted to put myself in the conversation, but I also wanted to be respectful, knowing how much attention and care Cameron brought to the position. I didn't want to tarnish the mark he had left. My next career move would not only give me the opportunity to gain longevity, but it would also set the stage for life as I know it today.

When things become difficult, appreciate the challenge. Be grateful for the pain, the tears, and the joy. Embrace it all because moments like this eventually turn into motivation.

Chapter 47

Create the Inclusive for Yourself

We all have to decide who we want to be at some point.

Society has a way of manipulating us into thinking we have to be a certain way, but it's not always how we see ourselves. Or how we want to be perceived by others.

Sometimes it's necessary to break away from the labels or roles we've been given. We have to see if there's something bigger waiting to be painted. If there isn't, we must learn to be happy living in between the lines society has created for us.

If there is indeed a bigger picture, however, there's an opportunity to do something bigger than ourselves. That's the moment when we control what we become – and do what needs to be done to ensure it aligns with who we are.

I've always wanted to be something bigger than myself. I watched my two brothers excel in karate class when we were growing up, as they both climbed the ladder to becoming black belts. I wanted to be part of a group as they were. I asked myself, *What if I could do something important?* and *If I could be a part of something bigger than myself, what would it mean in the long run?*

I didn't feel left out, but I thought I could find meaning in my life if I could be something bigger than my cerebral palsy. The sense of inclusiveness and belonging had been missing, although I never told anyone. I didn't like it, and wanted to change the way I felt. I thought it was just a phase I was going through and it would pass.

I didn't want to cause any trouble. Nor did I want to call any more attention to myself than my disability already caused. I was simply looking for some sort of validation that I belonged somewhere – and was capable of contributing to something. Several years went by and I was still watching my brothers climb the ladder at karate class – surrounded by their group of people.

I finally gathered the courage to tell my parents, *"I want to be something!"*

It took them some time to realize I wasn't talking about "becoming" anything. They slowly figured out I was looking for something much deeper.

I carried this mindset into my personal and professional life. It also meant, however, it affected my adulthood. It was just there at first, like a traffic light or a fly on the wall. It later occurred to me I needed to find out if this actually had a place in my life – or if it was extra baggage. If I dealt with this in a positive way, my decision to become a writer would mean even more.

I blinked and suddenly found myself in the final weeks of 2014. Things were going well with my career, and I was having more articles published by mainstream publications like Upworthy and XoJane. All those years of wanting to be involved in something big and important were coming full circle, but there was another vital piece to this puzzle.

I still had the opportunity to become the Social Justice Editor at The Good Men Project. It was a position my Editor and predecessor, Cameron Conaway, had brought relevancy and respect to. I wanted to make sure I did the same if I was going to even attempt to fill his shoes. I wasn't thinking about anything else as I replied to the e-mail regarding his resignation.

"It would be an honor to be considered for this," I wrote. "However, I understand if you have someone else in mind for the position."

I received a reply from the editing staff within hours, which stated they appreciated my willingness to step up, and the position was still open if I were to accept it. I wish I could say I wasn't taken aback, that I wasn't at a loss for words. Again, I was aware of the magnitude of this opportunity, but didn't think my name would be on the list of those who could possibly do what Cameron did, in the manner in which he did it.

I accepted the job with open eyes and a grateful heart. I understood how monumental this decision was – not only for me, but for the staff at The Good Men Project. I also understood this said something major about the way the staff handled business as an organization. My only goal at this point was to not let anyone down because I was finally part of a team. Even though I had been working at The Altoona Mirror for several years by now, my personal column did not give me the team approach I was looking for. That didn't mean I forgot about it or stopped writing it. I simply wanted more in my life.

There may be times when it seems like your moment will never come. A moment when you can breathe a sigh of relief in preparation for the task ahead. You might work hard and think no one notices – until they do. When that happens, it's your time to shine brighter than you ever have before.

Chapter 48

Up and Down the Peaks in the Valley

If there is no destination, there is no journey.

It's often that life is about the journey, not the destination. The journey has different peaks and valleys for each one of us, as does the destination. We learn to rise, fall, succeed and fail on our way to wherever we're going, but the lessons don't end there.

At some point, we have to realize a journey can't happen without a destination. Or at least an idea of where we want to be when the dust settles. We can only go so far before we hit a few bumps in the road. Sometimes, however, those bumps are so big and impactful they instantly put things into perspective, in a way that changes our world.

I don't think I could have been happier than I was at the end of 2014. I was at a point where I could enjoy life as a writer and genuinely think about my future. It was Christmas time and I found myself thinking about where I would be if I hadn't repeated second grade, been forced to drop out of college or made any difficult decisions along the way.

I don't think I would have been prepared to help other writers tell their stories. Or continue to send my work to mainstream publications while balancing a life outside of writing – one which still revolved around my cerebral palsy. I simply felt fortunate to not only be working on a regular basis but to also be building upon my career.

As I settled into my new role as Social Justice Editor at The Good Men Project, I started to realize this job – at least this part of it – marked the beginning of the rest of my life. It was an honor that I never thought would be bestowed on me – let alone help me grow professionally as well as personally.

It gave me a sense of peace. It wasn't the kind of peace that comes with knowing something is finished, like a painter putting final touches on a masterpiece. Nor was it a feeling of self-appreciation for going through the motions to even be in a position to help others. It felt more like breathing a sigh of relief, knowing I was truly moving on with my life in a big way. I didn't give much thought to what might happen if the rug was pulled out from underneath me – until reality threw a wild punch to my gut I never saw coming.

December 25, 2014 started out as a normal day. I woke up and finished some work from the previous evening, before heading upstairs to spend Christmas Day with my family. The smell of freshly baked cookies was in the air, our house was sprinkled with decorations and I couldn't remember feeling this happy, content and healthy in a long time – physically or mentally.

Everything was the way it was supposed to be – the way I've remembered it for so long. My family sat down for Christmas dinner and separated our gifts into piles according to the name tag on each neatly-wrapped package when we were done eating. We watched T.V. while opening presents from aunts, uncles and other relatives who live out of town. I quietly thought about all of the goals I had set so long ago, and how incredibly far away they once were.

It was a relaxing night. I admittedly needed to unwind and reflect. I went to bed shortly before midnight, feeling like I could conquer the world. The next morning, however, the clock seemed to stop and everything changed as I laid in my bed.

I reached down to uncover my legs and realized my sheets were soaked in sweat. My hand simultaneously brushed against my forehead. At that moment, I felt a rush of heat, unlike anything I've ever felt before. It was as if someone had lit me on fire. I knew something was wrong when I kicked my covers off – waiting for the immediate burst of cool air to hit me.

It never came. Neither did the feeling of control. I thrashed wildly in my bed – hoping to land on any spot on my sheets that wasn't drenched with sweat. With each tiny move I made, heat engulfed my body. I'd stop moving – trying to find some sort of internal balance. The moment I began to squirm or make any movements, however, the cycle started all over again.

This would become verbatim – a pattern that led to a cold, flu and many doctor visits. Two months and multiple tests later, in late February 2015, I was officially diagnosed with Graves' Disease by a thyroid specialist in Pittsburgh, PA. The disease – unbeknownst to me prior to this – causes extreme swelling of the thyroid due to an overproduction of hormones in the throat. Symptoms range from fevers and hot flashes to tremors in the arms or legs, in addition to being a very temperamental condition.

I can feel fine one minute. The next, however, it can feel like someone has their hands wrapped around my neck – enough that I physically feel pressure. Graves' Disease can also affect every major organ in the body – including the heart and liver. I wasn't sure how I felt after hearing the diagnosis. I was relieved to finally have concrete answers, but I was also more scared than I've ever been in my entire life.

There were moments in between the onset of Graves' and the actual diagnosis, where I felt like I was going to die. I had never been so ill, weak and depleted before – all in a matter of one day. I slowly had to learn how to live again and build myself back up from the very bottom. This time, however, I didn't just have my cerebral palsy to deal with on a daily basis. It was an extremely bitter pill to swallow – and it still is.

I still have Graves' Disease today, and I'm so grateful it's being somewhat maintained by the medication I now take every other day. That's not to say I'm accustomed to now living with a disability and a disease at the same time. I honestly don't think I'll ever get used to it, but I can't be sad and bitter forever.

My outlook on many things has definitely been heightened because of all of this. I'm much more aware of myself and being comfortable in my own skin all over again. The two months I spent looking and feeling like death were the lowest of the low, but feeling like I was in someone else's body only made me want to work harder to try to physically get back to normal -- or what I eventually came to recognize as *my* normal. The next few years would be a delicate balancing act on many personal levels – highlighted by receiving a prestigious honor in my hometown and the true realization of my lifelong dream: the publication of my first book.

It doesn't matter where you start out in life, or how long your journey takes. What matters is you find a light at the end of the darkest tunnel and follow it all the way to your destination.

Chapter 49

Crawl Out of Your Hole

Sometimes, we have to take a few steps back to truly realize what's going on around us.

Opportunity might be right in front of our faces, but we don't see it. Or we choose not to recognize a chance for success for one reason or another.

Maybe our situation causes emotional or physical pain. Maybe it brings us back to a bad place in our lives – or perhaps we don't quite know how to deal with our current circumstances. The part that sometimes gets lost in the pain and struggle, however, is everything eventually comes full circle.

These thoughts were so far away from my conscience in the first few months of 2015. My diagnosis of Graves' Disease took a very long time to pin down and had a tremendous amount of weight behind it. Not only was it a heavy dose of reality, but it physically drained the energy out of me like nothing else did before. it didn't help that my body temperature escalated at an alarming rate, as heat is a major trigger for Graves' Disease. Not only that, but I was wide awake every hour of every night. This is another clear sign Graves' had me in its grasp.

This vicious cycle continued for months on end, with regular doctor visits to Pittsburgh. I was a lifeless rag doll stuck in a skeleton's body because I was also losing a lot of weight, unable to eat, sleep or hold my head up – let alone write. It got to the point where I had to resign from my position as Social Justice Editor at <u>The Good Men Project</u>. I was barely meeting my deadlines at the other publications I was writing for, so I made the gut-wrenching decision to temporarily stop writing.

My body told me I needed to stop, but my brain told me otherwise. Months turned into years, and I was still struggling to function like a normal human being. Calls came pouring in from family members, who frantically checked in on me. They checked in with my parents every day, every week to see if anything had changed. I wasn't getting better, and everyone knew it.

When I lost the strength to write, I knew I was sick. It was a very clear indication that my case of Graves' Disease wasn't going away quickly or quietly, if at all. My symptoms were still strong enough to knock me down. I heard everything my thyroid specialist in Pittsburgh said – treatment for this would be long-term and the disease itself is extremely temperamental. In fact, I checked every single box off when I was given a list of initial symptoms upon arriving in her office in the dead of winter in 2015.

I had hit rock bottom, but I needed my own proof that things were as bad as my body was indicating. My inability to string a sentence together was all the proof I needed. As ill as I was, I reached a point where I had to come to terms with this. I had to accept the fact that my life had drastically changed literally overnight. Most importantly, I had to accept that I may never be the same again.

The next several years would be even more of a delicate balancing act. I wasn't getting better, but I wasn't getting worse, either. I had been taking thyroid medication long enough to somewhat stabilize the disease, but I couldn't feel a difference. I thought back to all the times I've had to fight – for myself and everything I've ever wanted. I also thought about my family and how they've always been there for me.

It was then I quietly decided I was done being sad, angry and whatever else I was feeling. It wasn't going to change the fact I had Graves' Disease. Nor was any of this going to magically go away. It was time to move on, even if it was inch by inch. The light at the end of this pitch black tunnel, however, would be brighter than I ever imagined.

I slowly started to come alive in the months that followed – eating, gaining the weight I'd lost and learning how to be myself again. Writing didn't come as easily, and I didn't expect it to. I built myself up to writing again because I didn't want to force it. I did, however, want to get back to the same level and quality of work I had before I got sick. Or as close to it as possible.

It was a very gradual, painstaking process – like crawling out of a deep hole. It was also something I was not prepared for. If I didn't make peace with what was going on, I knew I would be miserable. I needed to prove to myself that Graves' Disease wasn't going to get the best of me, even though it was the worst thing I've ever been through from a physical standpoint. And it still is.

I picked myself up as I began getting my life back on track, pouring my heart into every article I wrote and put my stamp on everything I sent out to publishers. I also dusted off the manuscript for my book of poetry and sent it out as well. That will always hold a special place in my heart because it was the blueprint for the theater production I directed in college – which became my senior project. I still wanted a chance to share the project with everyone all these years later. More importantly, I still believed there was a place for it in the world.

So, I submitted the manuscript to as many book publishers as I could. I was desperately trying to find some middle ground between being a writer and a patient with Graves' Disease -- constantly having to stop whatever I was doing because my symptoms would flare up. I'd let them run through me and then go back to writing. It became an exhausting routine, but I tolerated it because I had finally gotten strong enough to write again.

I continued to build myself back up, with the manuscript for my book floating around to potential publishers and the ongoing support of family, friends and my former professors at Penn State Altoona. It was June 2017 by now, and I was still doing whatever I could to get my manuscript published while balancing a plethora of deadlines. Little did I know, my world was about to drastically change again – this time with a letter from the staff at Finishing Line Press.

They were on the list of publishers I had sent my manuscript to, but I didn't think they'd send a personal reply back– especially after I'd been rejected by more than a dozen publishers. I held the envelope my mom brought down to my bedroom after getting the mail. I held it in my hand for a long few minutes – thinking, hoping and praying this was the break I needed to finally smash through the glass ceiling I'd been chipping away at for as long as I can remember.

It may feel like things will never change when you're in a bad place. You might not even be the one who put yourself there, but you're the one who decides whether or not to stay there.

Chapter 50

Dreams and Truth

Sometimes, the dream can lead you back home.

There are certain people whom we always want in our corner. It doesn't matter why we need their support or how many times we have to lean on them. We know they'll be there for us no matter what.

Then, there are those whom we hope will be there when we've achieved something great. Or when we reach a point where we can see – and share – the fruits of our labor. Maybe there are a few people who need some convincing that our hard work is actually paying off, or perhaps there's a handful of people whom we never thought would even give us a chance.

That's how I felt as I held the envelope from Finishing Line Press in my hand, on a hot summer's day in June 2017. I had a vice-like grip on it because getting it in the mail was so unexpected. My health, or lack thereof, became the focus of every thought and feeling I had. My symptoms from Graves' Disease were flaring up frequently and I knew when I needed to shut myself off from everything going on around me at any given moment. I also didn't know how I was going to feel from day to day, even though I had a small, yet strangely comforting peace of mind.

I admittedly wanted some good news more than I wanted anything else at this point in my life. I never thought Finishing Line Press might entertain the thought of publishing my small manuscript of sophomoric poetry. I had submitted the same manuscript into one of their annual contests several years earlier and was turned down. I assumed this envelope held the response for my most recent submission in 2016 – for the exact same contest I had entered before. However, I didn't want to let my hopes get too high.

In fact, I forgot I even entered this particular contest again, until my mom yelled, from the top of the stairs leading into my first-floor bedroom, "Erin, you got something in the mail from a publisher called Finishing Line Press!"

I wanted to believe this was the culmination of everything I've ever worked for. I wanted it to be proof I didn't spend the majority of my life chasing an empty dream. Most importantly, I needed a sign there was a light at the end of the tunnel I'd been stuck in. I took a few deep breaths while still clutching the envelope, nervously turning it over in my hand. My fingers touched the edge, ready to open it as my mom walked downstairs into my room.

"What's in that envelope?" she asked.

"I don't know," I answered. "I forgot I entered another contest a while back…"

I waited until my mom was sitting comfortably on my bed before slipping my finger under the open flap on the envelope.

I took another deep breath and slowly opened it and carefully unfolded the letter inside to read these words:

> "Thank you for your entry in our annual chapbook competition. Congratulations! Your manuscript has been accepted for publication in Spring 2018!"

I read a little further to find out I didn't win the competition, but Finishing Line Press had made the decision to publish my book in its entirety because of the quality of its contents. All I could do in this beautifully overwhelming moment was hug Mom as tears of joy rolled down my face.

I gathered myself before texting my dad – who was still at work – about a half hour later. I wrote, "I have something to tell you when you get home." I sent the text and tried my best to calm down enough to think or speak. I was so certain I was going to humbly add another rejection letter to my pile of failed attempts to get my book published. I was so sure this wasn't my time to show the world why I didn't give up on my dream, but my moment had finally come.

Later that night, my dad asked, "So, what did you want to tell me?"

I went into my bedroom and grabbed the envelope on my desk – with the acceptance letter inside – and handed it to him. He then asked what it was for, and what was in it. I told him it was a letter from a publisher, as he always checks with me to see if I have any good news. He put his car keys on the computer desk outside my room, sat down and opened the envelope.

He started to read the same words Mom and I had read earlier. At that moment, he stopped reading and gave me a huge hug without saying a word. I think it simultaneously hit all three of us that all my years of writing, editing and rewriting finally paid off. The proof was literally in my hands.

I began telling those closest to me the good news – friends, family and my professors from Penn State Altoona, who have allowed me to sit under their learning tree since Day One. As I went down the long list of names, I couldn't help but to think of my grandparents. I thought about what they would say if they could've been alive when my career truly started to blossom. Most importantly, I thought about what they both always said whenever they crossed paths with other people: "My granddaughter is the best writer in the world!"

Deep down in my heart, I believe their love and support carried through in every person who had a kind word to say about the impending publication of my first book. Being able to share this news with those who have been in my corner for so long, was more than an emotional moment. It was more than just getting good news and simply reacting to it. This was the culmination of every drop of blood, sweat and tears that has fallen on my keyboard for the better part of 20 years. It meant more than I can ever say.

It was tangible proof that I was meant to be a writer. Every hoop I've had to jump through was leading me to this. I felt unbelievably fortunate just to have the opportunity to finally become a published author. One phone call in January 2018, however, served as a very genuine reminder of where this all started.

> "Hello, Erin! I'm calling to inform you that you've been selected as the recipient of the 2018 WISE

Women of Blair County Award for Arts and Letters."

You might have a dream that starts in one place. You may even have goals bigger than your mind can contain at a given moment. Always remember where those dreams and goals begin. It will bring you back home when your journey takes you far.

Chapter 51

There Are Mountains To Move

We move them a little bit more each day.

Every day brings something new. It can be as small as waking up to see another sunrise – or as big as starting a new chapter in life. We often let hours pass before we decide to do something, only to realize there aren't any more seconds or minutes left in the day.

We tell ourselves we're going to start fresh the next day, but we sometimes look for excuses along the way. Things happen in the meantime – some we expect, others we don't. Some people might even claim we're not trying hard enough and we don't deserve the opportunities we get. At some point, however, we have to stop waiting and stop listening to all the noise.

I've never wanted to simply coast through life or ride anyone's coattails to get where I want to be. I've always wanted to live the best life possible, the way I was meant to. In the early months of 2018, I finally felt like I was on my way to doing just that. I was still trying to digest the fact that my childhood dream of becoming a published author was coming true, as I balanced my responsibilities at The Altoona Mirror along with the plethora of other publications I've had the privilege of writing for.

Living the life of a writer was no longer a far-fetched fantasy. The moment had come full circle, and it was one of the most indescribable rushes of emotion I've ever felt. I didn't have to ask which hoop someone wanted me to jump through. Nor did I have to question whether or not I followed the right path. In fact, there were several moments where I pinched myself leading up to the publication of my book – which has the same title as my senior project in college: *How To Wait*.

I realized the path I was on had never been paved before. I was making my own way through this part of my journey – and it was something I could truly call my own. That's why I was so shocked when I got the call. I had been chosen to receive the 2018 WISE Women of Blair County Award in Arts and Letters – an award presented to only one recipient each year.

The organization, led by a committee of strong, influential women in Altoona and Blair County, annually showcases other women in various categories, who embody empowerment and leadership in a business or philanthropic work in their community. The honorees are treated to a dinner on a special night in April, during which each one is recognized individually – in the presence of family, friends, local dignitaries and businesspeople.

I attended the ceremony in 2016 when one of my English professors at Penn State Altoona received the same award in Arts and Letters. It was one of the greatest honors of my life, along with being selected as one of the 20 most influential in Blair County under the age of 40 by The Altoona Mirror earlier that year as a part of their annual 20 Under 40 campaign. All of this unfolded before I knew about my book – and most personally, before I had something tangible to justify my claims that all I'd ever wanted to be was a writer.

I never imagined the tables would turn in such a beautifully unexpected way – one month before the release of *How To Wait*. My first thought when I heard I would be receiving my WISE Women award was, *What contest did I enter?* because I was entering so many in hopes of getting my work in the hands of editors.

I was in the parking lot at Penn State Altoona on a frigid January evening, coming home from a poetry reading, to find out a very close friend of many years had quietly nominated me for the award. My mom was with me that night and we both looked at each other in disbelief, as we tried not to scream with delight before getting in the car.

On April 18, 2018, I accepted my award from WISE Women of Blair County – surrounded by my family, friends, mentors, and faithful readers of my work. I joined an incredible group of women who, like me, want to spread a powerful message of empowerment and service within their local communities. Not only that, but I added my name alongside other women whom I respect and admire. It was a magical, surreal night I didn't want to end.

It did end, but the feeling of magic and empowerment held strong – all the way to May 4, 2018. It was publication day – the day I had been working toward and dreaming of for most of my life. I counted the seconds, minutes and hours until I could finally hold my first book in my hands, after months of getting frequent updates from the staff at Finishing Line Press.

I tried to distract myself while I eagerly waited for my first shipment of books to arrive. Nothing subdued my utter excitement, however. I went outside several times – hoping to catch the mailman before he got to my mailbox. The mid-afternoon sun was beating down on me, but I didn't care. I wanted to see my book.

I popped back in my house every few hours before deciding to stay inside and wait. Then, there was a knock at the front door. The sound of something gently being dropped on the porch followed. My mom opened the door to find a big box.

"This is pretty big," the UPS man said. "Can you sign for it, ma'am?"

"Yes," Mom replied with excitement. "I know what this is – my daughter has been waiting for it all day!"

My mom slammed the door and ran downstairs into my bedroom. She put the box on my lap and simply said, "Your dream has come true!"

We both tore the box open and found 35 author copies of *How To Wait* inside – neatly bound with a black and white picture of me on the front. I reached down in the box and pulled a book out. I felt as if I was holding a baby or a precious diamond. It was real. It was beautiful. It was perfect. Then, I saw my name – Erin M. Kelly – printed on the book and I burst into tears.

I couldn't speak or move. I was feeling every positive emotion possible, at the highest level. I just sat in my room and held the book to my heart. I quietly thanked every person I could think of before texting my dad a picture of me holding my box of books. For a moment, I forgot about my Graves' Disease or even cerebral palsy.

I have no one but the many people who have stayed by my side to thank. The people who saw something in me, and have been brave enough to help it grow and blossom.

I'm honestly still trying to wrap my head around living my dream all these years later, but I'd like to think of it as the equivalent of winning an Oscar. That's the only worthy comparison I can make now, or years from now. My hope for the future is everyone who's followed my career since Day One – or those who may have recently come across my work and find any worth in it – will continue on this journey with me.

If anything, I just want to say thank you. I'm glad you're onboard. The best is yet to come!

# # #

Forthcoming* by Erin M. Kelly

Erin's love of professional wrestling, her enthusiasm for life, and her passion for writing have created a perfect invitation for a friendship with the legendary Mick Foley. In her third book, Erin shares with her readers how this friendship came to be something that continually motivates her to enjoy life daily.

Subscribe to receive updates on this forthcoming, third book by Erin M. Kelly. Use the QR code below or go to:

https://bit.ly/MickFoleyBookByErinKelly.

Publication date TBD, most likely between Fall 2021 and Spring 2022.

Previously Published Components

This book comprises revisions of Erin M. Kelly's essays originally published by The Good Men Project.

1. https://goodmenproject.com/ethics-values/warning-storm-coming-wcz/
2. https://goodmenproject.com/ethics-values/abilities-outshine-disability-wcz/
3. https://goodmenproject.com/ethics-values/acceptance-delicate-thread-humanity-wcz/
4. https://goodmenproject.com/ethics-values/barries-dont-block-friends-wcz/
5. https://goodmenproject.com/ethics-values/the-never-ending-maze-of-life-wcz/
6. https://goodmenproject.com/uncategorized/perception-adoption-identity-wcz/
7. https://goodmenproject.com/featured-content/growing-up-around-men-wcz/
8. https://goodmenproject.com/ethics-values/trade-in-the-commodity-of-time-wcz/
9. https://goodmenproject.com/ethics-values/laugh-off-the-wall-wcz/
10. https://goodmenproject.com/ethics-values/get-goal-when-you-have-to-go-back-wcz/

11. https://goodmenproject.com/ethics-values/when-frustration-occurs-again-and-again-wcz/

12. https://goodmenproject.com/ethics-values/how-to-use-what-you-have-wcz/

13. https://goodmenproject.com/featured-content/the-measure-of-maturity-wcz/

14. https://goodmenproject.com/ethics-values/age-has-a-funny-way-of-changing-your-life-wcz/

15. https://goodmenproject.com/ethics-values/dangerous-delicate-power-wcz/

16. https://goodmenproject.com/featured-content/how-to-develop-a-quiet-respect-wcz/

17. https://goodmenproject.com/ethics-values/mutual-respect-showdown-wcz/

18. https://goodmenproject.com/ethics-values/trust-your-gut/

19. https://goodmenproject.com/featured-content/mindset-changes-rise-above-the-negative-wcz/

20. https://goodmenproject.com/ethics-values/life-throws-curveballs-when-we-least-expect-it-wcz/

21. https://goodmenproject.com/ethics-values/there-are-days-when-time-stands-still-wcz/

22. https://goodmenproject.com/ethics-values/where-are-the-loyal-wcz/

23. https://goodmenproject.com/ethics-values/worthwhile-moments-wcz/

24. https://goodmenproject.com/ethics-values/realize-the-potential-wcz/
25. https://goodmenproject.com/ethics-values/take-a-chance-on-yourself-wcz/
26. https://goodmenproject.com/ethics-values/theres-a-time-and-a-place-for-everything/
27. https://goodmenproject.com/featured-content/center-the-inner-force-wcz/
28. https://goodmenproject.com/ethics-values/lift-another-and-elevate-yourself-wcz/
29. https://goodmenproject.com/featured-content/burdens-to-bear-wcz/
30. https://goodmenproject.com/featured-content/momentum-motivates-wcz/
31. https://goodmenproject.com/featured-content/dig-deep-and-drown-out-the-noise-the-world-makes-wcz/
32. https://goodmenproject.com/featured-content/dont-let-them-tear-you-down-wcz/
33. https://goodmenproject.com/featured-content/finding-the-strength-to-let-go-wcz/
34. https://goodmenproject.com/featured-content/bounce-back-wcz/
35. https://goodmenproject.com/featured-content/clock-doesnt-stop-wcz/
36. https://goodmenproject.com/ethics-values/represent-yourself-and-let-it-out-wcz/

37. https://goodmenproject.com/featured-content/accomplishment-on-your-own-terms-wcz/

38. https://goodmenproject.com/featured-content/what-paths-life-takes-wcz/

39. https://goodmenproject.com/featured-content/the-lies-in-our-goodbyes-wcz/

40. https://goodmenproject.com/featured-content/vulnerability-is-a-scary-kind-of-magic-wcz/

41. https://goodmenproject.com/featured-content/when-the-stars-align-or-dont-wcz/

42. https://goodmenproject.com/featured-content/whats-worthwhile-to-you-wcz/

43. https://goodmenproject.com/featured-content/respect-rolls-the-dice-wcz/

44. https://goodmenproject.com/bits-and-pieces/be-the-moment-wcz/

45. https://goodmenproject.com/featured-content/the-fine-line-between-integrity-and-self-care-wcz/

46. https://goodmenproject.com/featured-content/appreciate-the-process-wcz/

47. https://goodmenproject.com/featured-content/create-the-inclusive-for-yourself-wcz/

48. https://goodmenproject.com/featured-content/up-the-down-and-peaks-in-the-valley-wcz/

49. https://goodmenproject.com/featured-content/crawl-out-of-your-hole-wcz/

50. https://goodmenproject.com/featured-content/dreams-and-truth-wcz/

51. https://goodmenproject.com/featured-content/there-are-mountain-to-move-wcz/

Subscribe to learn more about Erin M. Kelly and her writing projects, use the QR code below or use this link:

http://bit.ly/ResilientWriterWheels

Index

Awards..

    Top 20 Under 40..ix

    WISE Women of Blair County Award in Arts and Letters..ix, 188

Books...

    Bodies of Truth: Personal Narratives on Illness. Disability, and Medicine...ix, xi

    Disabled Monsters..viii

    How To Wait..ix, xi, 188pp.

    Man Box: Poems...ix, 202

    Praise Song For My Children: New and Selected Poems v, ix

    The Resilient WriterWheels..............................., ix, xi, 203

    To Cope and To Prevail...viii, xi, 134

People..

    Cameron Conaway.........................viiip., 143, 170, 202

    Dr. Ilse Rose Warg..viii, 134

    Dwayne 'The Rock' Johnson..1

    John C. Mannone..viii

Mick Foley..192

Mr. DeAntonio..58p.

Patricia Jabbeh Wesley...v, ix

Wilhelm Cortez..xiii

Places..

Korea..9, 18p., 22, 25

New York City..19

Penn State. ., 86pp., 92, 95, 99, 106, 108pp., 112p., 117, 119, 122pp., 127, 130, **134,** 157, 164, 180, 185, 188p.

Pennsylvania........................xi, xv, 19, 30, 86, 120, 139, 151

Shriners...30p.

Publications, Periodicals and Online Magazines..................

Breath and Shadow Journal..ix

Oberon Poetry Magazine..viii

The Altoona Mirror.........viiip, 120pp., 123p., 134, 137, 141, 149pp, 151, 155, 165, 170, 187p.

The Good Men Project. viii, xi, xiii, 143p., 147pp., 151, 154, 157, 165p., 170, 173, 178, 193

The Huffington Post..............viii, xi, 154p., 157pp., 161, 165

The Mighty...viii, xi

Upworthy..viii, xi, 170

Wordgathering: A Journal of Disability Poetry and Literature..viii

XoJane..ix, 170

Short Works by Erin M. Kelly (Essays and Poems)................

A Long Way from Hello..viii

Reluctant Reliance..ix, xi

The View From Here..viii, xi, 124

Also Published by Lasting Impact Press, an Imprint of Connection Victory Publishing Company

Listed in order of first publication date.

---

1. *How to Cope, Manage the Household, and Make Love When Your Wife Has Cancer: Practical Guidance for the Husband-Caregiver* by Michael D. Stalter, January 2016

2. *Curbing Human Trafficking: Sex slavery is a horrific international crime against women, men, and children. You can help stop it. b*y Mark J. Vruno, December 2017

3. *A Broken System: Family Court in The United States, Volume 1* by Stephen Louis Krasner, February 2018

4. *Man Box: Poems* by Cameron Conaway, April 2018

5. *Love 5.0: The Secrets for Being Close Yet Free and Having a Marriage That Lasts Forever* by Jed Diamond, Ph.D., April 2018

6. *How Did You Get Him To Eat That? 12 Parenting Practices That Lead to Healthy Eating* by John D Rich, Ph.D., June 2018

7. *My Distant Dad: Healing the Family Father Wound* by Jed Diamond, Ph.D., June 2018

8. Healing the Family Father Wound: Your Playbook for Personal and Relationship Success, by Jed Diamond, Ph.D. August 2018

9. *A Broken System: Family Court in The United States, Volume 2* by Stephen Louis Krasner, September 2018

10. Positive Parenting: A Practical and Sometimes Humorous Approach To Applying The Research In Your Home With Gender Inclusivity, Mutual Respect, and Empathy – and NO Spanking! By John D Rich, Ph.D., February 2019

11. Practical Parenting: A Workbook To Accompany Positive Parenting by John D Rich, Ph.D.

12. *tumbling: poetic thoughts from an anxious mind by* Elizabeth Joyce, November 2019

13. *The Resilient WriterWheels: Can't Is A Bad Word* by Erin M. Kelly, May 2020

Visit Connection Victory Publishing Company online:

http://ConnectionVictory.com

Made in the USA
Monee, IL
04 December 2020